University of Tehran Science and Humanities Series

Series Editor

Central Acquisitions Office, University of Tehran, Tehran, Iran

The *University of Tehran Science and Humanities Series* seeks to publish a broad portfolio of scientific books, basically aiming at scientists, researchers, students and professionals. The series includes peer-reviewed monographs, edited volumes, textbooks, and conference proceedings. It covers a wide range of scientific disciplines including, but not limited to Humanities, Social Sciences and Natural Sciences.

Mohammad Ali Besharat

Paradoxical Psychotherapy: A Practitioner's Guide

Springer

Mohammad Ali Besharat
Department of Psychology
University of Tehran
Tehran, Iran

ISSN 2367-1092 ISSN 2367-1106 (electronic)
University of Tehran Science and Humanities Series
ISBN 978-3-031-27716-0 ISBN 978-3-031-27717-7 (eBook)
https://doi.org/10.1007/978-3-031-27717-7

This Springer imprint is published by the registered company Springer Nature Switzerland AG
The registered company address is: Gewerbestrasse 11, 6330 Cham, Switzerland

Preface

Paradox refers to the clinical theories and practice put forward by Adler (1923), Dunlap (1928), and Frankl (1939). Adler (Dinkmeyer & Pew, 1979) and Kraupl Taylor (1969) described paradox as a positive use of patient's resistance against the therapist. In Dunlop's model (1928), paradox is defined as the process of gaining voluntary control over previously involuntary habits. Frank (1939, 1973) defines paradox as an existentially authentic distance between the patient and his/her symptoms. Bateson (1963) considers paradox as an inseparable part of the process of psychotherapeutic change. Haley (1963) and Watzlawick et al. (1974) believe that paradox is a technique for changing and correcting symptom-producing interactions among family members; which is described by Papp (1980) as some sort of imposing change on the family so as to preserve its coherence and integrity; the change that can happen through getting rid of present family models.

Pseudo-paradoxical and paradoxical interventions have been adopted and developed within the framework of different theoretical models, such as massed practice, stimulus satiation, implosion, and flooding in behavioral therapy (Allyon, 1963; Hall, 1943; Marks, 1970, 1972; Weeks & L'Abate, 1982), reframing in cognitive therapy (Mahony, 1986), paradoxical intention in Logotherapy (Frankl, 1939, 1991), and imposing change on the family in ordeal therapy (Erickson, 1959, 1964, 1965, 1973, 1977; Madanes, 1981; Papp, 1980; Watzlawick, Weakland & Fish, 1974). Paradox therapy has been further developed in various models of family therapy introduced by Milton Erickson (1959, 1964, 1965, 1973, 1977), Jay Haley (1963, 1984), Paul Watzlawick et al. (1967, 1974), Mara Selvini-Palazzoli et al. (1978), and Kelo Madanes (1981).

Along with theoretical and experimental developments in the process of knowing the therapeutic essence of paradox made by Adler (1923), Frankl (1939), Bateson (1955), and Selvini et al. (1978), there have always been obstacles and challenges to paradox therapy. These obstacles stem from five sources: (1) a total belief and faith in the incomplete doctrine of behaviorism and classical behavioral therapy (Dunlap, 1928; Marks, 1972); (2) incomplete and incorrect understanding of psychoanalytic theory and treatment (Crowe & Ridley, 2000); (3) defective and false prescription of paradoxical techniques (Crowe & Ridley, 2000; Mahoney, 1986); (4) superficial understanding of the influence mechanisms of paradox therapy (Akillas & Efran, 1995; Evans, 1980; Papp, 1980); and (5) moral issues and concerns about using paradox therapy (Doherty, 1985; Maranhao, 1984; MacIntyre, 1987;

Whan, 1983). On the other hand, psychoanalysts and the true practitioners and propagators of paradox therapy (e.g., Selvini-Palazzoli et al., 1978; Watzlawick et al., 1967, 1974) have never doubted the power, depth, stability, and effectiveness of paradox therapy. The healing power of paradox therapy, as practiced by Selvini et al. in Institute for Family Study, amazed Prof. Helm Stierlin and led him to admit, admiringly, to "the treatment of the patient and her family in less than an hour" (introduction to *Paradox and Counterparadox,* p. vii). This is undeniable clinical truth of families who have a member suffering from anorexia nervosa or some sort of psychosis, especially schizophrenia, reported in *Paradox and Counterparadox* (Selvini-Palazzoli, Ceccin, Prata, & Boscolo, 1978).

Beyond the different definitions of paradoxical interventions, clinical individual and family practice of paradox therapy, the moral issues of paradoxical interventions, and the theoretical bases of paradoxical models, the present work relies on more than 20 years of controlled clinical trials so as to introduce a model of paradox therapy that brings together different foundations, assumptions, and theories in a new order. The foundations and assumptions, as well as the way they have been brought together within a new psychotherapeutic model called "Paradox + Timetable = Cure: A perfect model of psychotherapy," have been given in "*Theoretical foundations of PTC: A perfect model of psychotherapy*." The present book, which suits PTC therapists, offers a complete report of the treatment process of 20 patients through which it discusses the practical aspect of paradoxical timetable, the prescription of therapeutic tasks and exercises, the management of each session, the effective mechanisms of paradoxical timetable, ending the treatment, relapse, and the roles of the therapist and the patient in the process of PTC. Beginning in 1998, the PTC model was applied for three years to volunteers visiting the University of Tehran Clinic, as a pilot. Since 2001, it has been taught in B.A., M.A., and Ph.D. courses in more than 40 terms and dozens of workshops around Iran. The sessions were videotaped for educational and research purposes, with the full permission of the patients. The patients were also asked not to take any medication or receive any other sort of treatment, psychological, or otherwise. In most of the cases, the patients arranged their sessions through the Internet, which made the treatment outcomes and follow-ups to be recorded in an orderly fashion. The report on the changes and the treatment outcomes were all carried out session by session, as well as the final assessments at the end of therapy. The possible subsequent visits and the follow-ups were carried out through the Internet.

The PTC model successfully applied to anxiety disorders, obsessive-compulsive and related disorders, and somatic symptoms and related disorders within a three-year period, first. Then, it was applied to other psychological disorders including personality disorders, couple and family problems, childhood and adolescence disorders, and certain types of sexual disorders since 2001 (e.g., Besharat, 2018, 2023a, 2023b, 2023c; Besharat & Naghipoor, 2019a, 2019b, 2022). The PTC model has been developed through 20 years and thousands of hours of therapy. It is a complete and special type of paradoxical therapy that has moved beyond the limitations and shortcomings of previous models and has produced unparalleled outcomes in individual, couple, and family therapy. The videos of all the sessions, taped with the patients' agreement, are available.

The present book aims to provide a succinct, yet comprehensive, practical guide to the PTC model. Most of the points referred to briefly in footnotes in this book have been fully discussed in *Theoretical fundamentals of PTC* (Besharat, 2023b). Some of the special and unique characteristics of the PTC model are as follows:

1. The PTC perfect model of psychotherapy is very easy, both for the patient and the therapist.
2. The PTC perfect model of psychotherapy is a very short-term treatment that is sometimes completed in two sessions.
3. The PTC perfect model of psychotherapy is a perfect and comprehensive model.
4. The PTC perfect model of psychotherapy is an economic treatment for the patients.
5. The PTC perfect model of psychotherapy is in line with moral standards.
6. The PTC perfect model of psychotherapy is a non-aggressive treatment.
7. The PTC perfect model of psychotherapy makes possible deep personality changes rapidly.
8. The PTC perfect model of psychotherapy decreases the use of medication to less than 20 percent.
9. The PTC perfect model of psychotherapy turns the patient into a therapist.
10. The PTC perfect model of psychotherapy decreases the chance of relapse to the minimum.

Tehran, Iran — Mohammad Ali Besharat

Acknowledgements

The PTC psychotherapeutic model is the upshot to years of clinical, psychological education, and experience, from my B.A. in Ferdowsi University of Mashhad (FUM) to my Ph.D. at the University of London. I should like to thank all my dear professors through these years. I have always been grateful to them. I especially thank prof. Mohammadmahdi Khadivi Zand of FUM. Professor Ivan Eisler was my supervisor for my Ph.D. dissertation at the Institute of Psychiatry, King's College, University of London. He was also the one who made it possible for me to have access to 68 videotaped sessions of family therapy of families suffering from eating disorders and to take part in a Four-year Systemic Family Therapy course at the Family Therapy Clinic of Maudsley Hospital. I thank Prof. Eia Asen, the head of Family Therapy Clinic at Maudsley Hospital, from whom I learned systemic family therapy and the use of paradoxical interventions in families. Professor Michael Crowe taught me couples and sex therapy within a two-year course. Professor Hans Jurgen Eysenck and Prof. Jeffrey Alan Gray were both great scholars who contributed immensely to the field of psychology. May they rest in peace! The PTC model is a synthesis of all the knowledge and experience I have garnered through the years and of course comes from working with all the patients who shared their priceless clinical experience with me. I wish to acknowledge their contribution both to this work and to the development of psychology and psychotherapy. I should like to express my deep gratitude to all of them, and I hope that our treatment sessions together have been able to help them become their own therapists, as is the purpose of the PTC model.

Contents

1 The PTC Perfect Model of Psychotherapy

The PTC perfect model of psychotherapy makes use of two basic components in dealing with psychological disorders. The first component, the paradox, means prescribing the symptoms of the disorder. According to this therapeutic technique, the patient (client)[1] must recreate the behavioral and the disorder symptoms, that is to say the same behaviors and symptoms from which he/she suffers and wishes to be cured of. In other words, he/she experiences them according to the tasks given to him/her by the therapist. The second component, the timetable, gives the patient a specific time and duration for doing the paradoxical recreation of the prescribed symptoms. The paradoxical timetable consists of these two therapeutic techniques. The two techniques must always be combined and applied together in the PTC model. The following are some examples of prescribing the paradoxical timetable to the patients.

The first example: Imagine a young, pregnant woman who suffers greatly from obsessive thoughts of torturing and killing her infant after it is born. The obsessive thought of child abuse occurs to her several times during the day, depriving her of her peace of mind. She has been so greatly harassed by these thoughts that she has decided to have an abortion in the seventh moth of her pregnancy, despite her personal wish to become a mother and her religious beliefs. She was told, over the phone, that she will be treated, and she does not need to have an abortion. The young woman gave birth to her baby, hoping that the obsessive thoughts would go away gradually. Her infant is now 45 days old, but the obsessive thoughts make her suffer stronger than ever every day and night. According to the PTC model, she is asked to recreate and re-experience the obsessive thoughts about child abuse at specific times during the day. The patient's daily routine and opinion are taken into account by the therapist, and she is prescribed three 5 min sessions during the day when she must recreate her obsessive thoughts. The patient suggests doing the tasks at 10, 17 and 22 (the therapist helps her in finding the best time). Her task starts from the day after her first visit to the therapist. She must find an appropriate place free of anything to bother or distract her and sit down, exactly on time (neither earlier nor later), to recreate the child abuse thoughts for 5 min. Within these 5 min, she must voluntarily summon those thoughts to her mind and visualize them with all the negative and painful emotions attached to them. The patient's responsibility is to make her best effort to do to herself voluntarily what the obsessive thoughts do to her involuntarily. In other words, she is on a theatrical stage, where she must play the role with which she has been living for a long time. That is why she can act well in it.

The second example: Imagine a young man who is compulsive with checking everything

[1] Words "patient" and "client" are used interchangeably in this book.

M. A. Besharat, *Paradoxical Psychotherapy: A Practitioner's Guide*,
University of Tehran Science and Humanities Series,
https://doi.org/10.1007/978-3-031-27717-7_1

several times. He checks the gas valve several times to make sure it is closed. When he wants to leave his apartment (or his office), he checks the computer, the light switches and the locks many times. After all this, he is still not satisfied and can't get rid of the doubts. The paradoxical timetable for this patient is as follows: at certain times during the day, he must voluntarily experience his pathological checking. Three 5-min occasions oblige the patient to check the gas valve, the light switch, the computer and the door lock several times. These checks are precisely identical to the ones imposed upon the patient, which he does involuntarily.

The third example: Imagine a patient suffering from excessive washing, who has been suffering from 120-min baths for six years. The disorder, which started six years ago, has gotten worse gradually and has, at present, disrupted her life immensely. Her suffering is not limited to the long bath, but begins before it in the form of fear of having to go through a fatiguing process of washing and not getting clean. Then, there is the severe stress of coming out of the bathroom and becoming dirty again. The best she has been able to do has been to increase the interval between the baths, which has become as long as a week at present. According to the PTC model, a paradoxical timetable is arranged for the patient. She is asked to choose a specific time during the day when she can wash herself up for 120 min in the bath. She chooses 19–21. Her task is, starting from tomorrow, to go to start her bath at 19. She is allowed to make it last as long as 120 min (the maximum time the patient stays in the bath).

I hope I have been able to give a general idea of how to prescribe the paradoxical timetable. There are, however, other points that need to be taken into account in this therapeutic model. I said that the patient must start his/her task from one day after he/she has visited the therapist. This instruction builds up the expectation that prepares the ground for the artificialization mechanism, which will be discussed later. Therefore, it is necessary for getting the optimum result. The patient is supposed to start his/her therapeutic tasks or exercises tomorrow. Will he/she be able to do them? What will happen during the exercise? What if he/she fails to recreate the negative emotions? What if he/she fails to do the exercise altogether? What should he/she do in case he/she misses an exercise for any reason such as oversleeping, not finding the right place, forgetting, etc.? What is he/she supposed to do at other times during the day? Should the patient do anything about the uncontrollable disease and the behavioral symptoms other than the tasks prescribed by the therapist? What is the therapist to do with the patient's surprise at this seemingly strange treatment method (the paradox)? How is he/she to respond to the patient's questions, concerns and fears?

Whether the patient asks any questions or not, he or she must receive relevant explanation from the therapist during the session and understand the process of treatment. These explanations are part of the treatment technique prescription. The therapist explains that although the task resembles a bitter medication, it is quite simple. "It is simple, because you have been experiencing it involuntarily for a long time and are therefore completely familiar with every aspect of it. You can play the role given to you better than anyone else. What you will do during the exercise may be even more complete than the explanation you have given to me, because you may have forgotten to tell me (the therapist) everything. There may be things you do not wish to share with me, or you may have skipped certain details. You must feel committed to do the exercise. You must prepare yourself on time, find an appropriate place, and recreate your symptoms and behaviors in all seriousness. You must make an honest attempt to make your exercise look as closely similar to what happens to you involuntarily as possible. You must recreate anything that bothers you, for which you have come here. This is all you have to do. Suppose you have been given a prescription to take a certain drug three times a day. Several possibilities might present themselves. The first possibility is that you manage to do the exercise on time, and recreate all the upsetting symptoms successfully, by about 100%. If you can do it, it's ideal. The second possibility is that you may not be able to do recreate all the painful emotions completely, but still manage to do it more or less, say by 50%. The third possibility is that you do your best, the similarity of what you do with your actual experience is close to zero. All these possibilities are fine, and you must not be worried about the difference between the task and the actual experience. As long as you make an honest effort, there is no room for worry. There is also a fourth possibility. You either forget to do the exercise on time, you are in a place where you cannot do the task or you are not alone. In such a case, that task is lost and you must not do anything to make up for it. You simply wait for the next turn. The reason is that these tasks are time-bound. In other words, you either do not do them at all, or you precisely do them on time. It also means that you are not allowed to change the time for doing the task, and shift it from 22 to 21:30 or 22:30, for example.

The therapist continues his/her explanations thus: "Another important point to take into account is that my prescription for you is to recreate and re-experience the behaviors and symptoms at the times we arranged together. I did not ask you to avoid anything (the symptoms), neither have I asked you to try to stop anything (the symptoms). You cannot do it. You have not been able to do it so far. If you were, you wouldn't be here. You just stick to what I have assigned you to do, and forget about everything else. Suppose you are not ever "there" at other times. This is the best cooperation you can have with me, and it's the best thing you can do to expedite your treatment. Next session, we can talk about what happens." Having received these explanations, the patient gets a general idea of what is supposed to happen. He knows what to do, and what not to do. All the possibilities are predicted and explained to the patient: he/she may succeed in recreating the pathological behavior completely; he/she may not succeed, or he/she may not even get a chance to do the exercise; the symptoms may or may not emerge at other times during the day. At times, the therapist may need to give one extra explanation to assure the patient: "Yes, I know that you are dealing with these symptoms, these obsessions, these behaviors and these repetitions 24–7, and you don't want them. However, according to the prescribed tasks here, you actually accepted that *you do want* to experience such symptoms and behaviors." This extra piece of explanation is given to those who have not been satisfied and have responded: "But, doctor, you ask me to do them three times for 5 min, while I'm dealing with them 24–7!" The therapist would say to the patient: Yes, you are dealing with the symptoms all the time but you don't want them. However, you accepted to deal with them voluntarily and willingly according to the arranged times here (say, three 5-min sessions during the day).

So far, I have explained how the paradoxical timetable is prescribed at the first session. There are some other points which will be discussed later on. The PTC model for psychological disorders is a very fast and short-term treatment method that requires a specific manner of interview the principles of which have been discussed elsewhere (see Besharat 2023a). The PTC therapist must be prepared to start the intervention from the first session. The clinical interview in this model focuses, mainly, on the patient's present complaint and its symptoms. The treatment process begins even without any diagnosis and identification of the nature of the disorder. This treatment is sometimes completed after a single session (which was the case about the patient one).

The usual interval between the therapy sessions in PTC is two weeks. The standard paradoxical timetable begins with three times a day. Even in cases diagnosed as severe by the therapist, it is still better to stick to the standard of no more than three times a day. Three is the sufficient number of sessions which gives the patient the opportunity to begin his/her treatment. The frequency of exercises decreases gradually. There are two weeks between the first and the second session. During the first week, the patient does the exercises three times a day. During the second week, he/she does them twice a day. In order for the patient to know exactly what to do (in the PTC model, the patient must always have clear-cut instructions), the times for both the first and the second week must be arranged during the first session. In the subsequent sessions, a new paradoxical timetable is arranged with regard to the improvement made by the patient. Usually, the same task is repeated with less frequency (once a day, and then every other day). This goes on until the patient is treated completely. In some chronic patients, this standard process might change, and the number of times increases gradually. It can be said that the dosage increases.[2] In such cases, when no improvement has been made by the second session (this is only in case the patient has followed the timetable closely- if he/she hasn't done the exercises, or has done them wrong, the same exercises are prescribed again) the tasks are prescribed for every two hours, up to the third session. If no improvement has been made by the third session, the dosage increases again and the tasks are prescribed to be done once an hour. On the other hand, if improvement is made from session to session, the frequency of exercises decreases. Three times a day becomes twice a day, twice a day becomes once a day, and so on.

The relatively standard interval between the sessions is two weeks. This standard has been defined through experience. Two weeks provide enough chance for the patient to do the exercises. Since the PTC model is a very short-time healing treatment, this interval gives the patient the opportunity to do the exercises and experience improvement, and bring him/herself to believe that real change is happening for him/her, despite the fact that he/she does not have to do the exercises all the time. There are plenty of times in which the patient does not do any exercises and he/she has the chance to see if the symptoms appear or not. Sometimes the therapist has to neglect this standard. For example, in case the patient lives very far from the clinic, goes on an unexpected journey or is on holiday, the interval between the sessions can decrease or increase without causing any problems. It is only important to remain faithful to the principles of the PTC model.

At the beginning of each session, the PTC therapist asks the patient to give a detailed report on the exercises and the possible process of change. The therapist must ask informed questions and lead the patient toward giving a thorough account of whatever has happened in the interval between the sessions. This is very important and helps the therapist and the patient to detect any possible mistakes and correct them. It also helps the therapist to trace the process of change and adapt further exercises according to it. Analysis of the exercises and the changes that occur from session to session, along with the proper interviewing techniques (Besharat 2023a), can strength rapport between the patient and the therapist, which is necessary for psychotherapy.

The therapists who have been newly introduced to the PTC model want to know two things immediately: (1) How many exercises should be prescribed for each patient? And (2) how long should the exercises be (based upon what criteria can one decide whether it is 5 min, 10 min or 15 min)? I have already given the answer to the first question. I will answer the second question after explaining the effective mechanisms of the paradoxical timetable. Before moving on to mechanisms, let us look at the treatment of three patients through the PTC model.

[2] Medical metaphors are used abundantly in the PTC model. This has several advantages including the simplification of the timetable for the patient, highlighting the necessity of doing the exercise on time, emphasizing the importance of sticking to the pre-arranged timetable, the simplification of doing the exercise through comparing it to taking drugs, preparing the patient to assume the role of the therapist (this is one of the characteristics of the PTC model which has been described under the titles of "Ending the PTC treatment" and "The relapse" in this book), and contributing to cultural normalization of mental disorders.

2 Client #1 (Female, 33 Years Old, Married)

2.1 Case Introduction

MS, a 33-year-old married woman, came to the University of Tehran Clinic complaining about intrusive thoughts related to torturing and killing her infant since the 7th month of her pregnancy. The thoughts have become worse since 45 days ago when she gave birth to her baby. The clinical interview based on DSM-5 (APA 2013), revealed that MS had the criteria for OCD. MS has put away knives and dangerous kitchen utensils because she is afraid that she might use them to torture her baby. MS has not had a history of psychological disorders and does not take medication at present. She has not received help from a psychologist or psychiatrist before and this is her first visit to receive a psychological treatment. MS was seen for 3 sessions over a period of 3 weeks.

2.2 Course of Treatment

Session One

Therapist (T): (After greetings and the social stage of the interview) tell me a little bit about what brings you here today.

Client (C): A couple of months ago, when I was seven months pregnant, I called you and told you it was quite a while since I started thinking about torturing my baby when he'd be born, and for that reason I thought of abortion. You said this problem could be solved and that you could help me get rid of these thoughts.

T: But you did not come for treatment then. You have come now that the baby is born. How old is the baby?

C: He is 45 days.

T: Is it a boy or a girl?

C: A boy.

T: Good. Do you still have those thoughts?

C: Yes. These intrusive thoughts hurt me really bad.

T: When did these thoughts start?

C: A couple of months before I had these thoughts, I'd watched a program on satellite television about child abuse. I watched and followed the program. In one of the episodes, I saw two mothers who told the story of how they beat their kids. One of them said she'd pull her kid's hair, the other said she'd slap her kid and burn parts of his body; I didn't have any problems in the subsequent days but the next week when a psychologist was talking about the problems of those two mothers, my problem showed up and since then these thoughts have been obsessing my mind. I always think I'd torture my baby when I'm alone.

T: Have you had these thoughts before you got married? I mean, when these type of thinking started in your life?

C: I had no thoughts about child abuse; I loved children so much and I even liked to work

M. A. Besharat, *Paradoxical Psychotherapy: A Practitioner's Guide*,
University of Tehran Science and Humanities Series,
https://doi.org/10.1007/978-3-031-27717-7_2

in a kindergarten.[1] When I pass by the newspaper stand, I'd like to read stuff about children, anything from child abuse to child psychology. Before I got married, I was a happy and cheerful girl but after the marriage, because of the struggles I had with my husband's family, I could not argue with them, so I always had this pent-up anger inside me.

T: How is your relationship with your husband now?

C: It's good. I have a good relationship with him.

T: Are you a happy couple?

C: Yes. But he doesn't know about this problem.

T: Didn't you tell him anything about it?

C: No I didn't.

T: Do you want to solve it on your own?

C: Yes.

T: I see. Are there any other problems?

C: You mean about child abuse?

T: Anything. About child abuse or any other problems. You said you might hurt the baby. Can you tell me how?

C: Just like those two women. One of them scorched her baby's body with skewers. The other one said she slapped the kid's face and pulled his hair. These thoughts come to my mind. I had to hide the skewers to prevent myself from using them but I can't get rid of these thoughts (in an emotional state, the client bursts out crying).

T: This is one of your problems. Are there any other problems besides child abuse?

C: No. That's all.

T: All right. I'll make a plan for you. It's very simple. You can do it when you leave here. The plan is easy but you should do it accurately. At certain times during the day, which we will decide about together, your task is to sit in a quiet place where you can concentrate and recreate all these thoughts for at most five minutes; I mean all the thoughts which have recently come to your mind unintentionally and you are familiar with very well. Based on my instructions, you should recreate these intrusive thoughts for at most five minutes and review them in your mind with all their sad and uncomfortable feelings; all those thoughts about beating, hair-pulling, slapping, throwing, and burning. All these thoughts have bothered you for months, but now, by following my instructions, you yourself should think about them at certain times of the day as if you are doing them to your baby. You should review these thoughts in your mind just like the time when you think about the scary scenes in horror movies.

There are some possibilities: First, you may do the tasks and recreate the thoughts very well and thus feel extremely sad. If this happens, you will have the best outcome very soon. Second, you keep on trying during the tasks but the thoughts come and go. There will be no problems. In Third, you try your best to bring the thoughts to your mind but they don't. Again, there will be no problems here because you did what you were supposed to do. The fourth situation is when you forget to do a task in due time (because of oversleeping or since the condition is not suitable) or when it is not possible for you to do the task in that particular time. There is no problem here either; however, you should skip the forgotten task and try not to do any other tasks to make up for it.

Now let's set 3 tasks, five minutes each. The tasks ought to be done on time, neither sooner nor later.

C: (With a little help and thinking) At 12:00, 17:00, and 22:00.

T: All right. (You won't have any tasks for tonight). You should start your first task tomorrow at 12 o'clock, the second will be at 17:00 and the last one will be at 22:00 at night. You

[1] This is an extemporaneous unconscious answer to the therapist opposite question! Saying that she loved children so much and liked to work with them in a kindergarten, expresses the tie between loving an object (children) in one hand and torturing the loved object on the other hand. These are wishes/impulses rooted in conflicts between the Id's drives and the Superego's demands. These are considered as natural and normal inter-psychic conflicts until the Ego is strength enough to manage them. The main purpose of the PTC therapy is to help the patient become strong enough to manage these kind of conflicts (i.e., ego-strength), like what is going to happen in this patient.

ought to do the tasks three times a day and continue them for three days. Later, it will be twice a day, what will they be?

C: 12:00 and 22:00.

T: Do these tasks till the next session.

Session Two

T: Welcome. In the first session, you were supposed to do some tasks. Tell me about them. What did you do and what happened?

C: I feel comfortable. I am so happy. I forgot three of those tasks.

T: You mean you forgot to do them?

C: No I did, but those thoughts did not come to my mind at all. I realized the next day that the thoughts never came to my mind. I felt well. There were days when the thoughts came but they were about those two women, not me. I no longer thought something was compelling me to do things to my baby. Once I thought about the woman who pulled her kid's hair and I burst into tears but I never thought about doing the same to my baby.

T: So what do you think about your situation in the last few days?

C: I feel so good. I don't know what happened but I'm very well.

T: The reason is doing the task. Hopefully the result turned out to be satisfactory. I suppose your problem is solved but I'll arrange another appointment so that I can visit you in a short session again. When you leave here, I'd like you to do the tasks twice a day for a week (at 12:00 and 22:00) and on the second week, you ought to do the tasks every other day, which will be on Saturday, Monday, and Wednesday.

C: Doctor, is it possible that the thoughts haunt me again?

T: I guess not. These thoughts will not haunt you anymore. However, we have enough time to see whether they come to your mind again or not. You have my instruction with you for the next two weeks and if you stick to that, they sure won't come again.[2]

Session Three

A day before the third session, the client let me know over the phone that she was not able to come and in a short conversation, it turned out that she was still feeling good and the obsessive thoughts no longer intruded her mind. The main reason for her refusal to come to the session was that she was upset that her husband might find out about her problem (a cultural issue).

2.3 Assessment of Treatment Outcome and Follow-Up

The course of the treatment was completed in 3 sessions. Assessment of the treatment outcome, which was based on the patients' comments in a graded scale of 0–100 and an open-ended question, indicated 100 percent recovery. A two-year follow-up evaluation showed no relapse.

[2]. In this case, the therapist briefly answered the client's question about the return of the symptoms. In some cases, it might be necessary to answer the client in more details. See the note under the title of "The relapse" in this book.

3 Client #2 (Female, 25 Years Old, Single)

3.1 Case Introduction

EH, a 25-year-old single woman, came to the University of Tehran Clinic complaining about fear of death. Fear of death had started in her about ten years ago, when she was fifteen. It had become worse and had disrupted the normal course of her life since a month ago when her grandmother passed away: "*For a month now, I've been feeling I'm about to die. This happens especially at nights. If I remain motionless for a minute, I feel that it's the end of me. I have to move my arms and legs so I can feel alive. Otherwise I die.*" Severe palpitations had made the patient to take Propranolol-10 every eight since a month ago. She had also visited the doctor at least once a week due to pains in her back and chest and had received tranquilizers to relieve the anxiety resulting from her intense fear of death. She checks her blood pressure every morning and every night, because she feels that she has a high blood pressure and may have a stroke. EH is living with her mother and her younger sister. This is her first visit for psychological treatment. EH was seen for 4 sessions over a period of 5 weeks.

3.2 Course of Treatment

Session One

Therapist (T): (After greetings and the social stage of the interview) tell me what brings you here today.

Client (C): I'm a kind of person who thinks a lot about death and stuff like that. After my grandma died, the fear of death overshadowed my entire life. During the last month, I felt as if I was dying, especially at nights. If I stay still for a minute, I feel like death is approaching me, so I have to move my hands and feet to feel alive; otherwise I might think I'm dead. I become short of breath from time to time and feel like I'm suffocating; my family believes that I make my condition worse and exacerbate the symptoms myself.

C: God bless your mother. When did she pass away?

T: In February (two months ago). But doctor, another relative of mine died before that, my father. I've experienced the death of my relatives before, but after my grandma died, this issue, the issue of death, became very important for me.

T: How long have you been thinking about death?

C: Since ten years ago when I was 15; but at that time the symptoms were mild.

T: When did you start worrying about it?

C: About a month ago. Doctor, I just sat and prayed and wished not to die (starts smiling). Life had become so horrible. I thought I had experienced nothing in this world. When I got out of the house, I thought everyone else had eternal life but God wanted to take my life right away. I thought something unfair was happening to me. It was awful, especially at nights. At nights, I thought I'd be alive as long as I was

M. A. Besharat, *Paradoxical Psychotherapy: A Practitioner's Guide*, University of Tehran Science and Humanities Series,
https://doi.org/10.1007/978-3-031-27717-7_3

awake and that I'd die if I slept. My eyes would burn so much because of the lack of sleep; but I just sat in front of the TV set until I got numb and only then would I sleep.

T: Let's get back to ten years ago when the symptoms were still mild, but were beginning to become more severe (which accidentally coincided with your grandma's death). What have these thoughts been associated with since then? What kind of thoughts, feelings, behaviors and symptoms were they associated with?

C: Doctor, I believe in dreams very much. I know that dreams are sometimes influenced by daily experiences. I know it, but when I see a dream and its interpretation turns out to be death, I freak out for a few days. Either I have to forget about the dream or I remember the death theme which makes me get mixed up. I'm not superstitious but I believe in dream interpretation, omens and stuff like that. These things have a big influence on me. I'd like to get rid of them but I can't.

T: Good! Is there anything else you might do to get rid of this situation besides being hard on yourself and staying up late at night[1]?

C: I can't doctor. I'm not able to.

T: Have you visited a doctor before?

C: You may not believe it doctor; I never visited a doctor before, but during the last month, I went to the clinic once a week around 10 or 11 o'clock at night. They gave me a tranquilizer injection because I felt my back ached so badly. I told them the pain was somehow related to my heart and I thought my heart would stop beating and my blood pressure would increase. I checked my blood pressure every day and night because I thought my blood pressure would increase and I'd have a heart attack.

T: What about other symptoms such as heart palpitations?

C: I take up Propranolol every eight hours because of the pounding of my heart. The heart pounding is horrible.

Some questions were asked about the family members (she lives with her mother and her younger sister), the interpersonal relationships, the client's personality traits, and the issue of whether her mother would be ready to come to the treatment session with her.[2]

I'll make a plan for you whose influence, in my experience, will begin a few days from now. I don't want you to stop taking drugs right away but from the next session, I'll ask you to do so. With the beginning of this treatment, you can stop taking drugs if you like. You don't need to, and you should not, go to any other doctors as long as you come here because it will interrupt our treatment process and it will do you no good.[3]

You have somehow described how worried you are about the subject of death but, you know, what you said is one thing and what happens to you in your daily life is another. You can't describe exactly how much pain you've been through, nor can the one who listens to you feel what really happens to you! According to the timetable that I'll draw for you, you need to do like this: at certain times during the day, you should recreate for yourself exactly what you have been experiencing for the last month. At these times, which should last no more than five

[1] In the PTC model of treatment before prescribing therapeutic techniques, the therapist needs to clarify some possible interventional experiences which the patient might have had beforehand. What has the patient done so far based on his/her own managements to solve the problem? Whether the patient has already received any professional help/treatment or not? The first reason for doing such probes is that the therapist must be aware of the patient's past interventional experiences. The second reason is that whether and to what extent these experiences have been useful according to the patient. And the third reason is that if the patient is receiving any other psychological and/or medical help? Leaving out all these arrangements and interventions before starting PTC and during the treatment is necessarily instructed to the patient.

[2] The PTC psychotherapy benefits both the foundations of systems theory and systemic techniques a lot. This book, as a basic practical guide for clinicians, however, is just limited to discuss the basic techniques of the PTC model. The systemic techniques of the PTC model can be seen in *PTC perfect model of therapy with couples: A practical guide* (Besharat, 2018).

[3] Both theoretical and empirical considerations of the PTC model require that a patient should not refer to different specialists simultaneously. Except in rare conditions, as a general principle of PTC, the patient should not be under any medication for the presenting disorder.

minutes, you should recreate and re-experience the fear and the thought of death as if you are going to die at that moment. I want you to recreate and live with the inevitable and unwanted thoughts and feelings which have been bothering you recently. You can do this recreation better than anyone else. In other words, I'd like you to play the role which you yourself have created; since you have been living with it for a while, you are more familiar with it and you know it in more detail than what you just described. In this regard, playing this role is not a difficult task. Doing this task may sound bitter to you but, you know, you have already had this bitter experience and you were not able to get away from it and you are experiencing it again and again against your will. In these tasks, you recreate and re-experience it on your own volition.[4]

You'll get the best result when you play this role as realistically as possible; if you do so, you may feel your heart pounding and the fear of death might terrify you. I hope that the recreation turns out to be just like what you experience in your life inevitably. If this happens we will receive the best outcome! But even if it does not, you can recreate the symptoms with any degree of similarity and that would be okay. There is another possibility; you might try your best to recreate within five minutes but nothing happens at all. If this happens, there is no problem because you have tried your hardest to do the task. Another possibility is that you might not be able to do the task within the due time for several reasons: you may fall asleep or perhaps you are not home or there might be somebody else around. If you happen to miss a task within a due time, you should skip the task then, and try not to make up for it. You won't do the task until next time. Let me put it another way: the task is either done within the proper time limits, which is arranged in the session, or it is not done at all.

Now let's draw a timetable according to which you should start the tasks from tomorrow. Think about 3 five-minute time frames within which you can do the tasks well. There should be regular intervals between the time frames when you are awake.

C: At 9:00, 16:00, and 23:00.

T: All right. Since you are about to come with your mother next week, let's draw the timetable for this week. Starting tomorrow, you should do three sets of five-minute tasks for the first three days (9:00, 16:00, and 23:00) and for the rest of the week, you should do two sets of five-minute tasks (16:00 and 23:00). Keep in mind that this is the only thing I want you to do. I didn't ask you to try not to dream, to stop believing in omens and dream interpretations or to live differently. I want you to remain the same person and in the next session you should be just like the person you have always been. You don't need to decide on anything and, please, try not to do anything special; and if you do so, it won't be of any use. You will be the same person tomorrow except that this task will be added to your behavior. Recreating the thoughts for three to five minutes does not mean that you should not have these thoughts and feelings at other times. You don't need to decide on anything or change anything. Please do not try to do anything more than what I said; it's not necessary to add or omit anything. See you next session.

Session Two

T: Welcome. Let's review the tasks of our first session for a few minutes, and then your mother will join us. So tell me what you have done during the last week. What happened?

C: I forgot to do one of the tasks for two or three days. At nights, I felt the same and there was no need to try to recreate it; during the day, I tried and sometimes it worked perfectly well and at other times it did not; the good thing is that I realized I was able to control the feeling when it rushed through me and I no longer feel the horror anymore but the thought of dying still remains.

T: So, you have occasionally done the tasks; at times the recreation turned out to be good but at other times it did not; at nights, the thoughts

---

[4] When prescribing tasks, the PTC treatment does not impose anything on the patient. All the tasks prescribed for the patients are exactly the same symptoms that the patient is experiencing in his/her daily life inevitably. This is the main reason that makes paradoxical timetable the easiest task in terms of the patient ability to do it.

are still present, but now the difference is this: although the thoughts have not gone away and are still there, they are not frightening anymore.

C: Yes, I thought I had them under control. They were just like a feeling[5] and they no longer had the horror of death with them.

T: How was your sleep during the last week?

C: Just like before. I had to get tired to drop off. Another thing that happened to me this week was that I felt I was not able to make plans for the next day. I thought I had no future before but now I think I have a future but I can't make plans for it.

T: It's been only a week since we started. I suppose your progress has been satisfactory. We need to continue. Now ask your mom to come; at the end of the session, I'll make plans for your next session (the rest of the session revolved around analyzing the relationships between family members, and getting to know the client and her personality traits through her mother's words.)

Your next session will be held two weeks from now. You should do the tasks during these two weeks like this: Do the five-minute tasks five times a day during the first week.[6] Last session, I told you how to do the tasks; you stick to what you did. Set five tasks, with five minutes for each. What time should they be at?

C: At 10:00, 12:00, 16:00, 21:00, and 23:00.

T: During the second week, you should do the tasks every other day (the client chose even days) and do them three times a day. At what time will you do them?

C: At 16:00, 21:00, and 23:00. Should I stop taking the drugs?

T: What did you do last week?

C: I used to take pills every night, but last week I took pills only for two nights.

T: So, till next session, it's up to you to stop taking the pills; but if you don't stop them by yourself, I will ask you to stop taking them from the next session. These pills have no effect on your wellbeing and you can stop taking them right now if you wish.[7]

Session Three

T: Welcome. Please tell me what you have done.

C: Doctor, I have done the tasks but I missed two or three of them during the last week. I did the rest, however, and the intrusive thoughts and feelings disappeared altogether. I had none of those feelings either during the day or at night.

[5] When describing their changes, the patients either refer to their ability to control the disorder or express new description of their symptoms completely different from the previous ones. For instance, "They were just like a feeling. They no longer had the horror of death with them", in the present case; "I felt like my head was getting cold, but it was over so soon and I felt no palpitations or difficult breathing or anything" in the patient #9 at session 4; "Slight thoughts just come and go, and I know they are nothing serious" in the patient #13 at session 8; "It's just like a wind which blows and goes away" in the patient #14 session 4; "They come and immediately go. They no longer stick in my mind to torture me" in the patient #18 at session 5; and "They come and go like shadows" in the patient #19 at session 4. Considering such descriptions give us a better understanding of the effective mechanisms of the paradoxical timetable.

[6] The process of increasing number of tasks, which refer to as increasing dosage in the PTC model, can be seen in explanation presented under the patient #12.

[7] Some points concerning why and how to cease medication are worth noting here. One of the principles of the PTC therapy is that the patient mustn't receive any treatment simultaneously, except in some especial conditions. So, any other intervention must be ceased. Within the broad spectrum of the anxiety disorders including OCD and related disorders, drug therapy has nothing more than sedative role. This is why the patients are interested and completely ready to cease medications not only because of their negative side effects, but also they are not curing. The process of ceasing medications would be different from one patient to another. The therapist warned the present patient at the first session that the medication must be ceased to make her ready for that. She then reduced her medications up to 70 percent in the interval between the first and the second session. Continuing the PTC tasks helped her to cease her medications completely by the third session! There was no need for the therapist to demand the patient to stop medications in the present case. The patient #3 presented by a different story. She had taken antidepressant medications for more than 10 years when started PTC. She had had the experience of ceasing/forgetting her medication for several times. The therapist suggested that she can do the exact way of ceasing the medications once more in the interval between the first and the second sessions while doing the assigned PTC tasks. What happened to the patient #3 in this regard supports the exclusive power of the PTC psychotherapy.

There were times when the feelings came but they were mild. I did not take pills at all.

T: All right. It seems that you have completed the personal tasks. Do you still feel upset like last month?

C: I don't feel terrified like last month.

T: You have stopped taking the pills. Have you gone to a doctor during the last two weeks?

C: Not at all.

T: How's your sleep?

C: Compared to last month, it's become better, but it's not normal yet.

T: Haven't you experienced waking up during the night and rolling over when you were sleep?

C: No I haven't.

T: I'll see you two weeks from now. During the first of these two weeks, you should first do the tasks for five minutes at night. Then you can get to sleep. And in the even days of the first week, you should do the task once a day (at 12:00). In the days of the second week, you don't need to do anything and in the even nights, you should do the tasks once just before you go to bed.

Session Four

T: Hello. Welcome. How's everything?

C: Fine. I don't have any problems. I think about death but it sounds normal and I'm not afraid of it anymore.

T: It seems that your condition has improved since you started doing the tasks and the thoughts and fears didn't come back to haunt you.

C: The problems I suffered from at nights no longer exist.

T: Have you stopped taking the pills?

C: Yes. I did stop taking them right from the beginning.

T: There are some thoughts, but they don't bother you. How's your sleep?

C: It's good. I can fall asleep very easily (starts smiling).

T: Now it seems to be the other way round (the therapist and the client start smiling). You don't force yourself to stay awake at night anymore, do you?

C: No.

T: Hopefully, the condition has been controlled. It will definitely not come back. You don't need to come into therapy sessions anymore. If you think you need to come here for any reasons, you can make an appointment and visit me again.

3.3 Assessment of Treatment Outcome and Follow-Up

The course of the treatment was completed in 4 sessions. Assessment of the treatment outcome, which was based on the patients' comments in a graded scale of 0–100 and an open-ended question, indicated 100 percent recovery. A 43-month follow-up evaluation showed no relapse.

4 Client #3 (Female, 32 Years Old, Single)

4.1 Case Introduction

Miss. MK 32 years old, single, was referred to the University of Tehran Clinic complaining about severe anxiety for which she had been receiving medication for more than 12 years. Based on DSM-5 (APA 2013), it was determined in the first session that the patient had the criteria for social anxiety disorder, including severe panic attacks in social situations and interactions as well as during exams. The main symptoms of the disorder included: rapid heart rate, extreme fear of a supposedly bad event happening, shaky voice, severe pain and spasm of muscles in the neck, shoulders and hands. The patient has had the anxiety symptoms since her childhood, however they worsened when she reached 13 and have intensified ever since. They peaked when she reached 20 and she had to take medication to alleviate them. The daily medication used by the patient includes Nortriptyline and Inderal 10 ml. Her family history shows that her mother and her two elder sisters had anxiety disorders too. This is her first visit for psychological treatment. MK was seen for 3 sessions over a period of 4 weeks.

4.2 Course of Treatment

Session One

Therapist (T): (After greetings and the social stage of the interview) What brings you here today?

Client (C): (the client starts laughing) I have an acute anxiety that has been quite relieved by medication. I never understood why it began in the first place. It manifested itself after a sudden anxiety attack ten years ago. It was during exams. Generally, I get extremely nervous during the exams and in academic situations. At that time, I was not able to attend the exam session and as a result I failed. I have been using different drugs since then but eventually Nortriptyline and Inderal showed good results. When I take Inderal, my heartbeat is controlled and my anxiety is reduced but when I don't, I become nervous and have trouble during my sleep. For instance, I forgot to take Inderal two days ago and as a result I became so nervous (It turned out that she first took high-dose Inderal but now she is taking 10 mg).

T: Well, what are the signs of this anxiety attack that you have been experiencing over the past ten years?

C: A racing heartbeat and an extreme fear of something bad that might happen. At the end, I imagine I've failed all the exams and have been expelled from the university. After all, I've always been the best student in the class but I think that was out of fear. I was afraid so I studied. Otherwise, I don't like studying. I am studious and I like studying a lot but when I'm being tested and I have to answer and speak, or during exams, I get extremely nervous. I always take Inderal when I want to give a presentation and if I don't, I get nervous, my voice shakes and I can't speak.

M. A. Besharat, *Paradoxical Psychotherapy: A Practitioner's Guide*, University of Tehran Science and Humanities Series, https://doi.org/10.1007/978-3-031-27717-7_4

T: Is this anxiety limited to exams, and presentations or does it happen in other situations?

C: Yes it does happen in other situations. I think I have a very low self-confidence in family situations and if I'm about to tell a long story in a family gathering, my heartbeat increases. However, if I am to tell it to a group of friends, I don't have any problems. For this reason, I think part of my problems can be traced back to my childhood and what happened at that time. The thing is that I've planned to study abroad for getting my PhD but I feel nervous and sometimes my neck and shoulders ache severely. Once I had cramp in my neck and my hand swelled and I had to go to a neurologist. They first said it was related to the cervical disc but when I received the MRI results, they said it was not related to the cervical disc but was a severe spasm. I constantly think when I go abroad, I won't be able to do anything. This hurts me a lot.

T: Well, you said you've had those anxiety attacks during exams. Were there other times when you felt the same?

C: For example, during the first session in the language class when I have to introduce myself, I get nervous and my heartbeat increases. I don't know why.

T: Well, seemingly this anxiety attack is not restricted to exams and grades. If you are about to speak in a group, say, introducing yourself, this condition exacerbates. Right?

C: Yes this is not limited to exams. When I'm about to ask a question in a formal setting, even though I receive positive feedbacks from others, I become nervous and my heartbeat increases. So I prefer not to ask any questions.

T: You talked about the racing heartbeats, the occasional cramps in the neck and shoulders and the pains in the muscles and hands which are somewhat controlled by medication, but still bother you. Did all these problems start ten years ago?

C: Ten years ago I started taking drugs but the problems were there since childhood. I remember when I was in the first grade, I happened to miss a point at math class. During the break, I rushed to my sister who was then in the fifth grade and burst out crying and my sister laughed and explained it to me, which was so simple. I have been such a coward since I was a little kid; I abided by the rules so as to prevent others from criticizing me.

T: You said you have been like this since childhood; what other experiences have you had?

C: Yes, I've been like this since childhood (clears her throat several times) but the problem of speaking in public started during the first year of middle school. In writing class, the teacher asked me to read my writing before the class (I was always worried about being asked to read my writing in front of the class). I remember my voice was shaking so badly and I could finish reading only with great difficulty. Since then, speaking in public has become a burden for me.

T: Let's suppose this problem stems from your childhood and has worsened since then. What other problems have you had up to now? What problem has brought you here?

C: The main problem is this anxiety.

T: Who in your family resembles you the most?

C: (The client gives a thorough account of the anxiety problems experienced by her mother and other family members).

T: So these conditions occur to you when you are supposed to take an exam or speak in a group. If we exclude these two situations, would this anxiety show up when you are alone or when nobody is around?

C: You mean even the thought of the exam isn't there?

T: You can talk about both situations, with or without thinking about exams.

C: I get nervous when I think about exams. When I'm getting ready for the exam, I feel nervous too.

T: What do you mean? Do you get nervous all through the day?

C: When I'm studying and getting ready, negative thoughts arise and make me think I won't be able to succeed.

T: So the treatment of your problem is limited to medication which you have been taking over the last ten years. Right? And at the same time, you are studying and getting ready for going abroad, aren't you?

C: Yes. And I've never been content with myself.

T: What do you mean by not being content with yourself?

C: I'm 32 years old now and I think I should have better conditions, but there are lots of incomplete tasks I haven't done yet.

T: The main issue we should deal with revolves around these anxiety states which should be treated. After the condition is controlled, you can then follow your plans. This aspect is part of your personal affairs which you can decide upon when you feel more relaxed. Now I should make a treatment plan for you. Can you put your studies aside for two weeks?

C: If you want me to, but currently I'm studying English.

T: I mean if you don't study for two weeks, will you be lagging behind or will you be able to make up for it later?

C: I will be lagging behind.

T: What if it's just one week?

C: I think I can manage one week.

T: Well, for the first week,[1] you just do the tasks I assign without any studying. During the second week, you should both do the tasks and study. That way, you will be able to compare the two situations better. It seems that you have taken the medication regularly.

C: I take my medication on a regular basis, but I have been sloppy too. I mean I forget a lot, but I always take the medication. If I happen to miss taking the drugs for two or three days, I feel bad and I start retaking them.

T: You did not skip taking the drugs on purpose, you just forgot to take them. What do you mean by being sloppy?

C: I don't usually forget things that are important to me. Forgetfulness and sloppiness are for the trivial or personal issues.

T: I asked you this because in my treatment plan for you, there is no room for taking drugs. You should not take the drugs for three days, just like when you forgot to take them before. The effect of our treatment will begin within three days and most probably you won't feel bad anymore. You can say goodbye to the drugs then. Now, pay close attention to what you should do from tomorrow on. You are supposed to do certain tasks according to my instructions. I'll explain a single task to you and little by little it'll be clear how many times you should do them and how.

C: Should I take notes?

T: No, it's very simple. You won't need to write anything. Each task takes 10 min and during this time, you are supposed to play a role. What role? The role of the person you are, which you have been playing during the past ten years. In your daily life, this role is inevitable and compulsory accompanied by the anxiety that you have described. Within these ten minutes, you are supposed to recreate these states exactly like the real ones with all the imagery, thoughts, feelings, behaviors, and bitter somatic symptoms. You have been playing this role for several years (of course it was unintentional and compulsory). There is no need for me to explain the role to you. You know it and can recreate it better than anyone else. The only difference is that now you play this role intentionally. You ought to recreate the scenes from the exam session, speaking in public and anything that can evoke the anxiety in you so that your heart starts racing and you feel the pain in your neck and hands, and the anxiety overwhelms you.

C: Should this role-playing have a scenario?

T: You can imagine that you are attending the exam session, or giving a presentation in the class or thinking about anything, in the past and present, that can make you feel more nervous. Everyone has his/her own way. The goal is to recreate the anxiety and stress symptoms within you exactly similar to what happens in your daily

[1] In the PTC model, the rule is to maintain the client's usual way of living and make the necessary changes within the context of his/her everyday life. This little change accepted by the client becomes necessary only if a) the objective encounter with environmental stimuli and conditions is not inevitable for the client and b) objective encounter with the environmental stimuli and conditions minimizes the fulfillment of "Ordering-artificializing" mechanism.

life, or even worse.[2] If that happens, it would be perfect. These tasks work like medicine, the only difference being that you buy the drug from the drugstore and take it, but here you make the drug yourself. You have to make the drug so that when you take it, all the anxieties arise within you even more severely than the usual ones.

C: Is it possible to create this much anxiety in ten minutes?

T: If you are worried that you might not be able to do the tasks in ten minutes, you can do them in 15 min. There is no problem with that. Ten is the maximum time limit, but if you realize that it's not enough, you can continue doing the tasks for 15 min. Now listen carefully. You try your best to play this role but it may not work out all the time. You may experience 50% of the real symptoms. There is no problem with that because you have tried your hardest. At times, you may not even experience the symptoms at all. Even so, there wouldn't be any problem because you have tried your best. Just keep in mind that if you can't experience the real symptoms at all, don't just sit there for 10 or 15 min. If you realize that nothing happens after two or three minutes in an assigned task, just leave the task and keep on doing your own work. Let me add that each of these conditions is acceptable only if you don't pity yourself, and only if you try your hardest to recreate the real symptoms by 100%. As I said, I want you to evoke the anxiety so well that your neck, shoulders and hands start aching and other symptoms arise. This effective treatment plan is the ultimate art of an actor playing a role.[3]

Another possibility that can occur is when you cannot do the assigned task on the due time; you may forget; you may not be in a proper place; you may have guests; you may be asleep. If you happen to miss doing the tasks on their due time, you cannot change the time of the task. You don't need that because if you miss a task, it wouldn't be a big problem. The number of tasks is enough to get the best outcome. Now, let's arrange three 15-min times during the day when you can do the tasks, starting tomorrow. The three occasions can be on any time, but they should be based on your current life circumstances. This way you are more likely to do the tasks. Compared to the rest of your plan, the first three days are very important since you won't take any drugs and won't do any studying during these three days.

After consultation and considering the possible times, the following occasions were agreed upon: 10:00, 17:00, and 22:00. It was also agreed that the tasks should be done twice a day on two working days of the week at 08:00 and 22:00.

T: The task should be done for 15 min on each occasion during the first week, and 10 min at the most during the second week. Keep in mind that the task ought to start from tomorrow. You shouldn't do any of the tasks tonight. You should quit the drugs from tomorrow and start doing the task. Another important issue is that you should just follow my instructions, and don't change anything. When I ask you to do the tasks on these three occasions, I don't want you to try to battle your anxiety at other times. You should just do your best of doing the tasks during these three occasions and you must not try to suppress or stop any feelings. Just do the tasks according to my instructions. At other times, the anxiety may or may not appear. Whatever happens, we will discuss it over the next session. See you two weeks from now.

C: Should I write down about what I do and what happens?

[2] These kind of expressions are impossible to be happened psychopathologically. These are just some supportive and encouraging expressions to maximize the possibility of "ordering-artificializing" (see "the effective mechanisms of the paradoxical timetable" in this book).

[3] The PTC therapist deliberately insists on such an exact recreation of the symptoms to provide the ground for the "ordering-artificializing" mechanism to be established. When the patient succeeds to recreate the exact involuntary symptoms, voluntarily, they are no longer exist as signs of the disorder. This therapeutic technique, which facilitates the process of treatment and makes it a very short-term therapy, is one of the PTC model characteristics.

T: No there is no need to do that. You will remember and tell me all about it.[4]

Session Two

T: Nice to see you. Please tell me what you have done.

C: The tasks were good; they were really effective. At the beginning, they were really effective, but they lost their influence gradually. If I didn't take the drugs for two days before, I wouldn't be able to sleep at all. But, although I didn't take any drugs during the last two weeks, I was relaxed at nights and I slept well. Now, however, I'm very nervous and I don't know why.

T: Do you mean right now?

C: Today I was so stressed. I don't know why. But it was very good. You asked me to try my best to experience the pains in the neck and hands but whatever I tried to contract my muscles, I couldn't and my muscles were even more relaxed. The pain was somehow eased (the client starts smiling).

T: You mean that what happened was the opposite of what you wanted, right?

C: Yes.

T: Did you stop taking the drugs from the first day?

C: Yes, I stopped them the day I left here.

T: Did you sleep well?

C: Yes, I did.

T: You said the tasks were more effective at the beginning, but later they were not. This is usual. By these tasks, you learned to experience a new way and the results have been satisfactory so far.

C: Yes.

T: This method could help you put aside the drug you have been taking over the past ten years. Now you are equipped with a method by which you can deal with and control the anxiety. Now by doing these tasks you can manage and handle the anxiety on your own without taking drugs. You said you were nervous today. This can be looked at from different angles. What I need to tell you is that all people become nervous. They are not relaxed all through the month. Any one of us can feel unwell. One may get a little bit nervous and the other may feel depressed depending on their personality differences. Your weak point is your anxiety and, like others, you are supposed to get nervous once in a while. The fact that someone may become nervous in life is inevitable and this can happen to and be experienced by everyone. The important thing is that, so far, you have been able to stop this anxiety attack quite well and later on, by continuing the tasks, you will be able to minimize the anxiety level and become normal. This normal condition disappears and the person's wellbeing decreases at times. This is normal and necessary in life. If everything happens as we wish them to, then we will become insensitive people. An insensitive person cannot feel what wellbeing is. Who can value a peaceful sleep? One who has experienced a disturbed one.

Apart from today, that you were not feeling well, how have you been during the past two weeks?

C: I've been better. I was called for a professional job interview. It was very stressful and I thought I had to take drugs to attend the interview. I just wanted to see whether I could handle it without any anxiety. It was very good. I was somehow nervous but I was not bothered. No debilitating anxiety got in the way when I was speaking (the client starts smiling).

T: Well, an obligatory event happened. It was quite risky.

C: (smiling) Yes, I thought so. But I couldn't check it with you. If I knew I shouldn't have gone there, I wouldn't have.

[4] Everything is taken place simple, brief, and fast within the process of PTC. The exclusive method of the PTC interviewing, therapeutic techniques, therapeutic changes, and the number of treatment sessions all are as simple, brief, and fastest as possible. In the PTC model of treatment, neither the therapist nor the patient need to take notes (except in rare conditions that the patient insists to write down some). Taking notes by the therapist within the treatment session will interrupt the rapport which is at the basis of any psychotherapeutic relationship. Taking notes prevent the flow of the interview, interrupt the extemporaneity of the patient's behavior (verbal and nonverbal), inhibit the genuine dynamic of the therapeutic relationship, and interrupt executive functioning of the therapist.

T: I wouldn't prevent you from going because I don't want to disrupt your daily life. I knew you have been waiting for their call for a long time. It's good that you have attended the interview, and the more important issue is that you have done a risky job which was too soon according to the treatment process, but the result was satisfactory. You managed to beat this arch enemy who has always defeated you and you were able to overcome it.

C: Most of the time they (the anxiety and symptoms of the disorder) didn't arise. You told me that sometimes I may not be able to recreate the symptoms, but it was more difficult and I could rarely recreate them. However, I was able to increase the anxiety for a couple of times. I have a blood disorder and I feel nauseous. At times, when I was able to evoke the anxiety, I felt nauseous. Generally, I think the task was very good. In fact, I am greatly interested now in attending your workshops and learning about this method.

T: You said that the nausea is related to the blood disorder. Why do you think they may be related to each other?

C: Because I have iron deficiency anemia and when it aggravates, my heartbeat increases and I feel nauseous.

T: I'd like you to think about this issue from a different angle. Look, there are many people who have anemia and there are many medical interventions for curing it and you can choose one of them. But I'd like you to look at it differently. Let's suppose it is rooted in your anxiety. We will put this feeling of nausea in our agenda and test it. If all or part of the nausea decreases, then it is suggested that the anxiety is the reason. If not, iron deficiency is the possible cause for which you need to go through the medical intervention. This is an opportunity and we can test it in the interval between the two sessions.

C: How?

T: I'll explain. Now you are equipped with an efficient method to tackle and control the anxiety. Before you used this method, the anxiety always dominated and defeated you like a powerful rival. You were weak, fearful, shaky and nervous which made the rival more dominant and fierce. You always wanted him to be away but he did not listen to you and wanted to be there and irritate and defeat you. Your inefficient behavior toward this rival was passive and avoidant. You never welcomed and asked him to be present. In this method, you welcomed and accepted him and wanted him to be present. Since you evoked the anxiety, it looks as if the rival were challenged and intimidated so he ran away. The rival learned that you are no longer afraid of him and realized that when you are challenging him, you have a lot to say. Before that, the anxiety debilitated you but now you are debilitating him and since you seriously asked him to come, he vanished into thin air. The first possibility that we talked might happen would be perfect and would knock the disorder down. I provided you with this explanation to let you know what actually happened so that you can more ready to add the task about nausea to the other tasks.

It's necessary to continue the tasks for another two weeks. Within these two weeks, the treatment process will be completed. We will finish the treatment plan next session and then I'll explain what you should do later on. During these two weeks, you should do the tasks twice a day, each lasting at most ten minutes. (C: on regular days at 10:00 and 22:00 and on working days, at 08:00 and 22:00). Recreate the symptoms like before for the first 5 min and add the task for nausea to the second 5 min. I mean you should try to feel nauseous and throw up. Keep in mind that if you feel nauseous at other times during a day, don't stop it because, as I said before, you are not supposed to stop anything.

Session Three

T: Hello, nice to see you. Tell me what you have done in the last two weeks and what happened.

C: In the last two weeks, I was only able to do the tasks twice. I couldn't do the tasks as regularly as before. I tried very much but it didn't work. I became restless and I couldn't do it. However, I was able to do it a couple of times but they were not serious. It looked as if what I was doing was useless and I didn't have any problems with it anymore.

T: You mean you were not able to do the tasks anymore, because there were no problems, right?

C: No they weren't.

T: You said you were restless. What do you mean?

C: I wanted to stop. I was bored.

T: Can we say you were bored during the tasks and not at other times?

C: Yes I was bored only during the tasks. I was okay at other times. Last time, I did the tasks well. Sometimes my anxiety increased and sometimes it didn't. However, this time the tasks themselves were annoying and I don't know why I was bored with them (the client starts smiling).

T: In other words, the tasks became unpleasant and you didn't like to do them. Have you been well for the last two weeks?

C: Yes.

T: Did you continue to improve?

C: Yes. I had been quite nervous during the first two weeks but during the second two weeks, I wasn't nervous at all.

T: What about nausea?

C: I felt nauseous at times but I think that was because of my stomach. Because of the strict diet, I had to lose weight and this weakened my stomach. Whenever my stomach is empty, I feel nauseous.

T: Your experience tells you that the nausea is related to your stomach, right?

C: Yes. I'm sure.

T: Well, I thought it might be related to your anxiety and decided to test whether this hypothesis was true. Now, you are telling me that these two issues are not related to each other. Your experience might be true. Probably these two issues are not related.

C: Doctor, I'm worried that the problem might return.

T: it's normal that you are worried. Everyone might become worried. Now let me explain to you about this concern and the possibility of a relapse. This is the last session in our treatment plan. You will go out and live your life perfectly well. Based on my previous experience, I guess that the problem will not return. Now, let's suppose that the problem will come back. What should we do? You are now equipped with a method which acts like an ointment for injuries. The injury is healed but the rest of the ointment can be used later on if it's needed. You have been in this condition for years. Now, you are worried that the problem may return. If the anxiety returns, just wait for five days to see whether it lingers or not. If it disappears within five days, just do nothing because it may return for a day and disappears automatically. However, if it stays and lasts longer than five days, simply make a treatment plan just like the one we made before and follow it. Make tasks and do them three times a day on certain occasions, with each task lasting ten minutes. You can keep this prescription to you for a rainy day.[5] However, you are always welcome to come to the clinic if you need help.

4.3 Assessment of Treatment Outcome and Follow-Up

The course of the treatment was completed in 3 sessions. Assessment of the treatment outcome, which was based on the patients' comments in a graded scale of 0–100 and an open-ended question, indicated 100% recovery. A 3-year follow-up evaluation indicated that there was no relapse.

[5] Self prescription (self therapy) is one the simplicity aspects of the PTC treatment model. Possibility of the relapse must be taken into account as a part of the psychotherapy process. Therefore, it must be discussed by the therapist at the end of the last treatment session, even if the patient doesn't be aware to ask for it. The therapist explains when and how the patient can prescribe a paradoxical timetable for him/herself as he/she has already learned and experienced during PTC. Such ability reduces the necessity of more treatment sessions, lowers the treatment expenses, and the most importantly promotes the role of the patient as a therapist (also see notes under "The relapse")!

5 The Effective Mechanisms of the Paradoxical Timetable

5.1 Introduction

How can the paradoxical timetable treat the patient immediately and decisively within the framework of the PTC model? What happens to the patient that treats him/her? Are the therapeutic changes in this method superficial or deep? Is the treatment permanent or temporary? To answer these questions, we need to learn more about the effective mechanisms of the paradoxical timetable. The paradoxical timetable creates therapeutic changes through four mechanisms, as follows.

5.2 The First Mechanism: Ordering-Artificializing

The truth is that disorders and their symptoms, from the point they emerge in a person as the result of certain conditions to the point when they reach the serve their purpose, are neither artificial nor obey orders. The therapist uses controlled time (timetable) plus the disorder itself (paradox) so as to prescribe exercises for the patient (order) through which he/she can recreate and re-experience the symptoms according to a plan (artificial). The symptoms may emerge (become active) in one of two ways: they may emerge contrary to the patient's liking and fulfill their function, which is to cause pain and discomfort to the patient; or, the patient may be able to activate the symptoms and experience them whenever he/she wants. When this second scenario presents itself, the patient has been successfully able to turn a natural phenomenon into an artificial one. This new, artificial phenomenon, is only superficially similar to the natural, and therefore pathological, disorder.

In line with the therapist's orders, the patient must do his/her best to make the artificial symptoms as identical to the original ones as possible. However, this is impossible and can never happen. Only a similarity in terms of appearance is possible. There are several reasons for this. To put it simply, within the framework of this mechanism, the disease or disorder is neither artificial nor obeys orders. It does not comply with the patient's will, and does not come and go as the patient wishes it to. It is called a disease precisely when it is beyond the patient's volition, comes and goes as it pleases and is, therefore, painful to the patient. Whatever is under the patient's will is not a disorder and does not have anything in common with the disorder.

The philosophy behind arranging several times (e.g., three times a day) for doing the paradoxical timetable is that the process of artificializtaion can occur. Determining a specific time for doing the exercises allows the patient to use his own will and freedom to recreate symptoms. The more the exercises are, the less likely it is for the natural and the artificial symptoms to correspond. When the patient takes the first step successfully and experiences artificial symptoms, the second mechanism is activated.

M. A. Besharat, *Paradoxical Psychotherapy: A Practitioner's Guide*, University of Tehran Science and Humanities Series, https://doi.org/10.1007/978-3-031-27717-7_5

5.3 The Second Mechanism: Breaking the Link between the Symptom and Anxiety

Once the symptoms have been recreated and re-experienced artificially, the patient faces a new phenomenon, experience, and reality. The symptoms are there, but they do not have the bitter anxiety usually attached to them. When a behavior or symptom does not cause anxiety, it is no longer pathological. It has become quite useless. Thus, the link between the symptom and the anxiety is broken. The advantage of the PTC model is that it removes all the anxiety (that is at the core of psychological disorders) attached to a situation immediately and without inflicting any pain on the patient. The central principle in the PTC model is the removal of anxiety. Any therapeutic approach that can omit anxiety can be considered a successful and practical approach. The healing art of the PTC model is that it expedites the process of anxiety reduction and removes it in a simple practical way. The PTC therapist must take this principle (the minimization and removal of anxiety) into account through all the stages of the treatment. When the patient reports, after doing the exercises, that the symptoms of the disorder are no longer painful to him/her, it means that the link has been successfully broken. When he/she says that the symptoms have started to sound foolish, it means that the link has been broken. When he/she says "I felt the symptoms were so childish, and I simply didn't do them anymore", it means that the link has been broken. "Before some exercises, I kept telling myself that I must remember to do the exercise. But, quite surprisingly I still forgot them," means that the link has been broken. When the link between the symptom and the anxiety is broken, the bitterness of anxiety, which is fed with emotions, affects and feelings, goes away. A new phenomenon takes its place: the meaning of the symptom is changed. This is the third mechanism.

5.4 The Third Mechanism: Changing the Meaning of the Symptom

Before the therapeutic changes started, the symptom reigned over the psyche of the patient as an undisputed opponent, a disaster, an incurable plague, an infinite torture, a ceaseless stress and a never-ending disease. The PTC model turns all these meanings on their heads. When the interview and the treatment begin, from the point when the patient is instructed to recreate the symptoms and live with them, the meaning of the symptoms changes for the patient and for the system (usually the family) surrounding him/her. From now on, the symptoms are valid and permissible. In fact, they have to exist (symptom prescription) and the patient (and the system) looks positively at their existence within the paradoxical timetable and experiences them voluntarily. This cannot be true about symptoms that were formerly described as domineering, undisputed and never-ending. Now, they have lost their previous meaning. In the next stage, when the paradoxical timetable is carried out, the symptoms can no longer equal disaster, pain, torture and anxiety. They have found new meaning. In this new equation, the patient (say former patient) has the upper hand over the condition, and the symptoms no longer even exist in order to be called the defeated opponent or the former malady. This special change in the meaning is the result of the PTC model. The more the disorder loses its negative meaning, the more the patient is able to form a stronger self that cannot be shaken easily. This is the fourth mechanism: the ego-strength.

5.5 The Fourth Mechanism: The Ego-Strength

Relying on psychodynamic paradigms, especially Freud's tripartite model of Id-Ego-Superego, and taking into account a different view of the superego and the interaction among these tree fundamental structures of the psyche in the PTC model, it is necessary to give a brief account of this triangle and its role in mental disorder and health. Id is the biologic and innate capital for every individual which is born with him/her and is the source of two drives: life and death. These drives are called aggressive and sexual drives when talking about individuals and personality traits, as well as in psychopathology and psychotherapy. Ego is another structure that takes shape gradually, as the person amasses experience, and equips itself with tools and skills that help it fulfill its role as the executive manager of the personality. A major part of the energy of ego is spent on solving the continuous conflicts between the id and the superego to create levels of balance between the two. The superego emerges as the oedipal conflict reaches its summit, the aggressive drives toward parents are repressed, the sexual drive toward the parent of the opposite sex is curbed, and identification with the parent of the same sex come into existence. The superego inherits oedipal conflicts, stems from the id and receives its capital from it. Therefore whatever id does, in terms of eating, drinking, mating and killing, has a parallel in the superego in terms of preserving, caring, warning, preventing and avoiding. These two old opponents have a conflictual relationship with one another. One pulls downward while the other aspires upward. They would not tolerate one another and fight constantly if the ego does not come between them. They are like siblings that fight childishly all the time and need the motherly role of the ego in order to put in their place. An authoritative ego between the id and the superego can both satisfy their needs and resolve their conflicts. Mental health exists under such a condition. If the ego is weak, the siblings go wild and make a mess. Mental disorders appear in this case. Therefore, the strength of the ego determines whether the individual is healthy or not. But, how does the PTC therapist invigorate the ego?

The process of ego strengthening can be better understood through an example. Suppose two world champions in wrestling must compete against one another in the final of the Olympic Games. The two world champions are highly experience wrestlers who have been opponents for a long time. Who wins the game? Before the game begins, experts predict, based on the wrestlers' background and present conditions, that the blue wrestler will defeat the red one. The red wrestler, hoping to win the gold medal, tries to keep his spirits up. But he cannot help feeling that he has no chance against the blue wrestler. The game begins. The mental atmosphere is in favour of the blue wrestler. The red wrestler is wrestling under a lot of stress. Suddenly, the blue wrestler makes a mistake and the red wrestler gets two points. It all happens in just a second. What do you think has happened in the minds of the two wrestlers? The red wrestler has regained his confidence. He will not let his distressed opponent to get the two points back that easily. The two wrestlers have switched psychological roles. Now, the blue wrestler is the underdog. The red wrestler has taken the situation in hand. He feels brave and has lost all his fears. This new situation gives him the opportunity to control and defeat his opponent.

Let's go back to the example of mother and the noisy brother and sister. If the mother has authority, she knows that the children are noisy and playful by nature. Therefore, she does not expect them to behave unlike their evolutionary nature and allows them to play. However, she defines rules and principles that serve as a framework that prevents chaos and disorder. The authoritative mother pretends she has not seen some of the mischief done by the children. Also, the children realize that there are limits to what they can do and that they are not allowed to surpass those limits. When the mother leaves home, the children find a perfect opportunity to do whatever they want at home. The minute they hear their mother coming back, however, they put everything in its place and try to restore order. The mother knows what has happened, but she pretends not to notice anything (and the children feel relieved). Everything is in order and health is maintained. What does a weak mother do? Or, what do children do to the weak mother? Whatever they want! They do their duty, as if they have been born to raise hell. Now, what if somebody comes along and helps the mother become more authoritative and adopt the right method of dealing with her children? Again, health is restored.

The PTC therapist is the benevolent helper. He helps the patient deal with his problem. When conflicts between the id and the superego take the form of pathological symptoms and anxiety, they can upset the ego. If the helpless ego resorts to the paradoxical timetable to deal with the conflicts, it can break the link between the symptoms and anxiety, take control of the situation and teach the naughty children a lesson. Once the ego gets the golden points, it does not lose them again. It's vital health dictates it to take hold of the points no matter what happens. It should be mentioned here that this deep structural change guarantees the stability of therapeutic change and decreases the possibility of relapse (i.e., the weakness of ego after its strength).

The process of ego strengthening can happen fast and even suddenly, or gradually. The prior level of ego strength, which is different in every one and is a function of the individual's former life experience and personality differences, is the main factor in determining how fast this process occurs. The coach trains all the players equally. But not all of them can get the gold medal. Some reach standards sooner than others. This is out of the coach's hands and is determined through the players' individual differences. This is the main reason why the length of treatment differs for the patients receiving the PTC psychotherapeutic method. However, such individual differences do not prevent the therapist form doing his/her job. In other words, the PTC therapist does not evade responsibility for the immediate treatment of the patient and looks for ways of making it happen as soon as possible. The first and the second complement are two techniques that help the therapist along the way.

5.6 The First Complementary Technique

The PTC therapist is ready, from the very first session, to conclude all the session with assigning exercises the patient must do till the next session. This short-term psychotherapeutic model does not waste some sessions on classical interviewing the patient. The report given by the patient in the second session is conclusive. The improvement made by the patient, and the percentage he/she gives, shows us how successful our player has been in the field, to what extent he/she has been able to do the exercises, how accurately he/she has managed to carry out the technique and how strong his/her opponent is. Suppose our OCD patient takes baths as long as 120 min, and we intend to decrease it to 30 min. It is normal for the PTC therapist to expect the duration of the baths to have decrease to 60–90 min by the second session, and to 40–50 min by the third session. In the end, he will reach the optimum 30 min. If improvement is not made somehow in this manner, we have two choices. First, the situation dictates us to give the patient a larger dosage of exercises (look at the discussion about increasing the dosage in the report of patient # 12). The second scenario is different and does not necessitate increasing the dosage. Suppose the patient has done his/her tasks well and has made an acceptable improvement by the third session (40–50 min baths). However, he/she expects his/her baths to decrease to 30 min as fast as possible. This expectation corresponds to the patient's wishes, but does not correspond to his clinical reality and the process of treatment. More importantly, it can increase the danger of stress in the middle of the treatment. As we said before, the principle ruling over the PTC model is decreasing/removing anxiety. Therefore, the therapist must intervene immediately and prevent the anxiety from going up again. How can this be done? The first complementary technique comes in handy here. The patient is told that it is necessary to keep his/her baths at 60 min for some time. Decreasing the duration any further would have negative consequences for him/her. Offering an explanation that sounds convincing to the patient can be useful here. Here's an example: "You are now like an overweight person who has lost too much weight in a very short time, and it is bad for her health. Therefore, she must decrease the process of losing weight." The patient is asked not to try to take baths shorter than 60 min. This instruction removes the extra anxiety and paves the way for decreasing the duration further. In the PTC model, the first complementary technique is usually used from the third session on, and not before the third session.

5.7 The Second Complementary Technique

Sometimes, the first complement does not suffice and the second complement may be needed. Remember the patient who couldn't decrease the duration of his/her bath to less than 60 min after the third or the fourth session. He/she is full of anxiety and expectation. Maybe the first complement does not help us attain our goal. The best it does is to decrease the bath to 40 min after two more sessions. Under such a serious clinical circumstance (that can be influenced by the patient's other conditions, severity and duration of the disorder, all of them, or other reasons) it is necessary to prescribe the second complementary technique. The PTC therapist asks the patient to try to keep the 40 min and do not exit the bath any sooner even if he/she can. It is almost as if the therapist and the condition have switched places. Similar to the condition, the therapist would like the symptoms to stay and keep torturing the patient. The patient cannot believe what he/she hears. Under this amazement, and oblivious of concerns about the treatment outcomes, anxiety is disarmed. There is no place for anxiety anymore. Anxiety for what? When the anxiety is not supposed to become less, why should the patient be worried about it not having decreased? So far, the patient has been worried over what would happen if the anxiety does not decrease. Now, he/she must not allow the anxiety to become any less than what it is. One of the orders given by the PTC therapist at the very beginning of the treatment process, irrespective of whether the two complements will be necessary later on or not, is that if the symptoms intensify for any reasons during the treatment, the patient is not allowed to make attempts to decrease them. And this is another principle governing the PTC model. If we feel the need to give the patient more explanations, we can go back to the weight loss example. "You have lost a lot of weight in a very short period of time, and now, you need to gain a little weight so as to avoid any other problems". The rationale behind prescribing the second complementary technique is in line with the central principle governing the PTC model: decreasing/removing anxiety.

6 Client #4 (Female, 44 Years Old, Married)

6.1 Case Introduction

Mrs. FH, a 27-year-old married woman, came to the University of Tehran Clinic with her husband. They married 23 years ago and have three children. The clinical interview based on DSM-5 (APA 2013), revealed that she had been suffering severe OCD. The main OCD symptoms included frequent doubts about prayers, repeating endless prayers, and repeating specific religious rituals before prayers. Her OCD started 6 years ago with a little bit different symptoms which later on focused in religious ablutions and prayers. The religious compulsions have become worse since last year leading to personal and family problems, especially within the couple's relationships. Her husband has also become more and more impatient and critical toward her. FH has not had a history of other psychological disorders and does not take medication at present. She has not received help from a psychologist or psychiatrist before and this is her first visit to receive a psychological treatment. FH was seen for 4 sessions over a period of 5 weeks.

6.2 Course of Treatment

Session One

Therapist (T): (After greetings and the social stage of the interview) Tell me why you are here.

Client (C): Thank God I have a good life, I have good children, and my husband has been very understanding of my problem through the past six years. It's all about my prayers. My problems showed themselves through prayers.

T: What happened six years ago? What was the problem, and how it affected you so much that it made you come here?

C: It started as some sort of compulsion. If I wanted to sit down on a sofa, I had to put a piece of paper beneath me. Nobody could touch me. When I got out of the bath, not even my youngest child could come to me. Everybody was at their wit's end, and I was the worst. If my hands were wet, I had to wait for them to dry. In the bathroom I washed and scrubbed my hands and my legs so hard. I couldn't sleep on the carpet without having something to lie on. I have become a little better since then, but my obsessions with saying prayers gets worse and worse every day.

T: So, you didn't have any obsessions about prayers at the beginning, right?

C: That's right, at first it was all about cleansing, and saying prayers became an obsession later on. Now, I am full of doubts when I say my prayers. I use some signs during my prayers, which I follow so as to be able to say my prayers through to the end. Nevertheless, sometimes I doubt whether I've already done some parts of the prayers or not, and I have to start the whole prayers again. I really don't know what to do.

M. A. Besharat, *Paradoxical Psychotherapy: A Practitioner's Guide*,
University of Tehran Science and Humanities Series,
https://doi.org/10.1007/978-3-031-27717-7_6

Husband (H): Sometimes, she says her prayers over and over again.

C: Now, I keep feeling I haven't done Wudu[1] properly. It is not actually so, but since I feel doubtful, I have to do Wudu again.

T: So, you stop saying your prayers …

C: No, no. I don't stop it. I say my prayers through completely. Then, I feel I haven't done something right, so I do Wudu and prayers again. There are times when I do this up to ten times.

T: Do you do Wudu for every round of prayers?

C: Yes, I do. And I usually do Wudu several times before getting ready for each prayers.

H: (Sarcastically) I would like to know why you do Wudu several times. My stomach made noises, she says. What has that got to do with anything, I say? She doesn't eat anything lest her stomach should make noises.

C: I don't eat anything before two to three hours before saying prayers.

H: She knows it's all right. I keep telling her, you're the only one who can help yourself. I go check whether she says her prayers right. I tell her she has done it the right way, but she insists on doing them again. I have been trying to help her for the past five, six years.

C: I believed what he said before, but I can't anymore. I've gotten accustomed to it. When somebody talks to me for the first time, I accept. I know it all, but I can't accept the word of people around me anymore.

H: We can't take trips anymore. If we want to go to a party, it has to be after the even call for prayers, when she's said her prayers. She has to take a shower every morning, do Ghusl[2] and other rituals and say her prayers.

C: I have to do Ghusl every day.

T: You mean you must do both Ghusl and Wudu for your prayers?

H: She feels she is impure.

C: I'm always torn with doubt. Therefore, I feel that I'd better do Ghusl before saying prayers. I have to be absolutely clean. I don't trust myself anymore. I can't even talk to my husband like a normal person. If I talk to my husband, I have to do Ghusl before saying prayers!

T: You think that you've become impure through talking, and you have to do Ghusl, right?

C: That's right.

T: How many times a day do you wash up?

C: Once a day, sometimes twice a day. I definitely take a shower in the morning. Sometimes, after a nap at noon, I wash up again. I think that since I was asleep, it might have become necessary for me to do Ghusl.

T: There is no shower between the prayers, and it's just repeating Wudu and prayers several times?

C: No, there is no shower, there's just Wudu and prayers.

T: At present, you take a bath once or twice a day, and do Wudu and prayers several times?

C: Yes.

T: What else?

C: Well, for example, I've been invited to a party for next week. I become distressed. I keep worrying about taking a shower and being able to say my prayers right so that I can get to the party on time. I am a total psycho. It's easy to say, but God knows what torture I go through.

H: Sometimes, she starts crying during her prayers.

C: I cry after prayers. I cry over my problems. I don't how I ended up like this. I feel sorry for myself, I keep asking why me? I look at people around me. They all say their prayers, probably without doing what I have to do at all. I ask myself, why can't I be like them?

T: Since six years ago when your obsessions started, what changes did it go through? Has it remained unchanged, has it increased or decreased?

C: It has increased every day.

T: What happened to the compulsions about touching others, or sitting down?

H: They have decreased.

T: But they are still there?

H: Yes. To give an example: I reached over to remove a strand of hair from her dress. Why did you touch me after having just touched your shoes? She protested. And the dress wasn't even the one with which she says her prayers.

[1] Ritual Islamic purification before saying prayers.

[2] Islamic ablution.

T: Right. Have you visited any specialists for this problem over the years?

C: Not a specialist, but once I had a cleric pray for me, and since I believe in religion, I was great for about fifteen days. We were rebuilding parts of our house then, and the noise did not bother me at all. Oh! (describing her present conditions) I also have to unplug the telephone while saying prayers; I must turn down the TV. I have to make sure nobody comes while I'm saying my prayers. If my son is outside, I call him and ask him to come back in no sooner than an hour, so I can finish my prayers. I can't invite guests over. We can't invite my daughter and son-in-law. I can just get one week of rest every month, when I don't have to say prayers. I do everything, such as parties and guests, within this week.

T: You mean the week you are on your period, right?

C: Yes. That is the only week I'm relaxed.

T: You don't have to say prayers one week a month. What happens to other issues such as taking baths and the cleaning during that week?

C: None. I feel completely at ease. I don't care about anything. I know it's all because of prayers.

H: At other times, if the neighbors make noise, if she hears a car horn, if somebody rings the bell or whatever—things that are totally unrelated to her—she thinks that her prayers are not acceptable anymore.

C: That's right. I feel palpitations whenever I decide to say my prayers.

H: She cannot breathe.

C: I say my prayers with such haste and panic. I feel I'm dying of anxiety and stress. Sometimes, I really feel bad.

H: Her problem is only with the prayers.

T: What else have you done for your problem?

C: Nothing. I called religious references several times and asked religious questions.

T: Did it help?

C: Not at all.

T: How long does it take you take a bath?

C: (Laughing!) It is really ridiculous. Sometimes, I do Ghusl up to 10 times when I'm in the shower and it's still not enough. I keep telling myself, let's do it one more time. One more! And the water is running and being wasted, which I know is a sin.

H: (Sarcastically) Well, let me ask you this: what kind of Ghusl do you do?

C: Ghusl Janabat.[3]

H: But, Ghusl Janabat is not required in such cases.

C: Well, I feel it is.

T: Let's suppose Ghusl Janabat has become obligatory for you three days ago. You did it then, and Ghusl Janabat has not been necessary for you ever since. But you do it anyways. Your husband wants to know why you do it. You answer that you feel the Ghusl you did three days ago was not done properly, is that right?

C: No. I feel that maybe something has happened when I was asleep. I do the Ghusl again because of my doubt.

T: Therefore, there is no actual reason for you to do Ghusl Janabat. You even believe that the Ghusl you've already done has been done correctly. But you have doubts that maybe something has happened in the meantime that makes Ghusl necessary for you.

C: That's right.

H: Or, suppose she is talking to me. If there is a slight discharge of fluid she does Ghusl Janabat. (Sarcastically) Now, I would like to ask you: what kind of Ghusl is that?

C: Well, I need to do the Ghusl to make myself feel better.

T: How many times do these Ghusls happen, and how long does it take each time?

C: Sometimes, I do them up to 15 times. And they don't take long; about 15 min.

T: Does it take 15 min from the time you start your bath to the time you finish it?

C: Yeah. It takes about 15–20 min. This is because I do the Ghusl so fast, because I'm stressed. I say my prayers really fast, as well. I think that I recite all the words and verses correctly, but others tell me I do them too fast. I do it fast, because I don't want to be worried over whether I've recited them right or not.

[3] This kind of Ghusl is done after sexual intercourse and/or having an orgasm.

H: (in a critical tone) Doctor! One of her faults, which I've told her about multiple times, is that she just repeats Arabic words one after the other like a parrot. She can say ten prayers by the time I finish one. She just parrots them. Saying them like that doesn't mean anything, I tell her. It's better to say your prayers only once, but to understand the meaning of what you are saying.

T: Daily baths happen once or twice, about 15–20 min each time; and you do Ghusl 15–20 times. Is that right?

C: Yes.

T: How long does it take you to say your prayers?

C: If my husband is home, he doesn't let me to do it in longer than 30 min. But if the obsession overcomes me, it may take 2 h, or 2 h and a half.

T: When do you say your prayers?

C: It's important to me to say them on time. If I don't say them on time, I'll really be sick. I get so stressed that I can't take it anymore.

T: You say all the 5 daily prayers right on time?

C: Yes. I only do the morning prayer without Ghusl, because there is no time for taking a shower. I just keep hoping that I've done it right. But I still have to make up for it later on when I do Ghusl, because I keep thinking that the prayer might not have been acceptable.

T: Does this only happen with your morning prayers?

C: Yes. This is because I don't have enough time in the morning. I say the other prayers so many times that I start to feel satisfied.

T: How was it for you before six years ago, when it all started? Were there any problems, then?

H: There was no problem at all. We were so happy. I don't think there is anything wrong in her life. Thank God we have healthy kids, I keep telling her. We have no problems. You're living in comfort. I treat you well. I always pamper her, doctor. I really love my life.

T: Does anyone in your family have a similar problem?

C: No. They all make fun of me. They tell me I should be ashamed of myself. They think it's wrong.

H: Her mother, who is my aunt, is a very religious person. But even she doesn't do what my wife does. She says a lot of prayers, but she does it according to religious demands, not disproportionately.

T: How about her father?

H: Her father is also religious, but not as much as her mother. I think she's taken after her mother.

C: My mother wants me to benefit from the religious rewards of saying prayers. So she keeps telling me to do it.

H: I' really tired of her prayers. There are times when our children must go hungry for two hours before she finishes her prayers and prepare the meal. I got so exasperated the other day that I took away her Turban and prayer rug. Then I found a note in her drawer asking her to recite one thousand Salawats.[4] Some of what she does is recommended to her by her mother. She has enough problems without you telling her such stuff, I tell her mother.

T: Well, let's move on. How is your relationship as husband and wife?

H: I think it's absolutely perfect, and good. I can't stress this enough. When I go to work, I keep looking at my watch. I can't wait to finish my work so that I can go back home to my wife and kids. I want the time to pass as fast as possible when I'm outside, and to freeze forever when I'm home. I really love my family. Really! (addressing his wife) What about you?

C: Me too. When my husband leaves for work, I can't wait for him to come back. If he is late, I call him. When he's home, I'm calm. I get stressed and nervous less frequently.

T: Well, have the problems you told me about influenced your sexual life as husband and wife? I want you to compare your life now with years ago when everything was still normal.

C: It has definitely influenced our relationship. I suggested that we make a plan for that, instead of doing it randomly. And he accepted.

[4] Religious salutation upon the prophet of Islam.

T: Has it helped to improve your relationship?

C: Yes, we have totally solved our problem in that respect.

T: How frequently do you have sex?

H: We agreed on twice a week.

T: And do you both enjoy it?

C: Yes, it's according to the plan. And I have no problem with it.

T: Do you take medication?

C: Not at all.

T: How old are your children?

C: My junior son is in the fifth grade. He is 12. My older son is 17, and my daughter, who is my first child, has been married.

T: All right. I am going to explain to you what we will do. So pay close attention. First, you need to correct your understanding of the problem, and then we will make a timetable for you. One of the symptoms of this problem, as you explained yourself, is that it is some sort of obsession. The person suffering from it knows that her doubts are baseless and wishes that she can say her prayers and do other religious rituals normally, like everyone else. She suffers from her condition more than anyone else. But she can't help it. She would like, very much, to not have such a problem. But the problem is imposed on her and she cannot escape it. It's not like she wants to be like that. It's not like she doesn't want to get better. She does want to, but she can't. I want you to pay attention! She wants more than you, her husband, and more than anybody else on the face of this earth to not have this problem. But she can't help it. It's out of her control. She likes to be able to say her prayers normally, just like you. But obsession overcomes her, and fills her with doubts about everything. Her judgment and reasoning tells her that she has done her prayers and her Ghusl right. But obsession creates such an immense doubt in her that she cannot comply with her reasoning. The obsession makes her to repeat things over and over again. You, her husband, can overcome any doubts that may come to your mind concerning your prayers or other religious rituals. You simply suppose that you have done it the right way. But as for her, obsession doesn't let her take things easy. Therefore, the problem here is neither lack of knowledge or willingness; it's simply lack of the ability to change. That is why anything that religious references say about prayers can't and won't influence her behavior. Because they have said things she already knows. She has heard them from the religious references before, and learned them by heart. She actually abided by them before the obsession. They are not saying anything new. They can't give any practical help for dealing with the obsession. Therefore, whatever they say won't change anything. Why? Because the lack of ability to change is still there. The problem is this lack of ability.[5]

It's simply beyond her ability to change. (addressing the husband) Take yourself for example. With your present height and weight, you can lift 20 kg. But, can you lift 100 kg? You certainly would like to do it, because you will get a medal for it. But you can't. Do you think it would be right if I keep telling you to try harder or to do your best? It's definitely not right. I explained all this because I want you to stop having irrational expectations of one another. Don't reproach one another on account of the problem that is beyond your ability to solve. She likes, more than anyone else, to prepare your meals on time. She likes, more than anyone else, to say her prayers right and on time. But she can't. She doesn't need us to teach her such things, since she knows them already. She doesn't need encouraging, since it is her greatest wish to be able to change. It is only that she cannot change. I want you to remember what I just said, since it is necessary for your treatment. What we try to

[5] One of the assumptions in PTC is that the persistence of dysfunctional symptoms is due to the inability of the patient rather than his/her understanding capability. This assumption, along with the other assumption in this model (i.e., the foundational role of emotions and affects in developing and perpetuating psychological disorders), require the therapist to always remain within this principle; respect the patient's sense; avoid sedative techniques; avoid instructional/educational teaching; and keeping the paradoxical-timetable treatment clear of cognitive misconceptions. Cognitive doctrines and rational reasoning lack the force and the efficacy of healing emotional experiences.

do here is to enable her, step by step, to regain the ability to change.[6]

So far, you have led a specific lifestyle. When you leave here, you follow along the same path with some minor changes that I will ask you to make. In the following week, you will live as you have always lived. Of course, I mean about the compulsive washing, Wudu, Ghusl and the prayers. I am not talking about the rest of your life. You will just add to your daily routine the timetable that I will give to you. Therefore, when you leave here, you are not supposed to try to change or reduce your compulsions. Do as many prayers as you think you need, just like yesterday. Just like yesterday, do Ghusl for several times. I don't ask you to do anything different at all. You will just add to the rest what I ask you to do. I repeat for the last time: you will reduce nothing of what you have always done.

First of all, when you leave here, (addressing the husband) you must not interfere in the obsessive prayers and Ghusl at all. You must not comment on what she does, neither is she allowed to ask you to give your opinion or supervise anything. You have nothing to do about the problem while the treatment is being done. You must not ask for advice or help from anyone else, be it close relatives or friends. Just follow my instructions and orders. You (addressing the wife,) already know when you must say your daily prayers. Can you also tell me a specific time for taking the daily showers?

C: I take the first bath at about 10:30–11:00, and in case I feel I need a second one, I do it at 16:30–17:00.

T: Starting from tomorrow, you must add an extra series of prayers and showers to the ones you routinely do every day. To put it more clearly, when you finish saying your actual morning prayer, say another morning prayer as my prescription. Do the same about the later prayers throughout the day. Repeat whatever for the extra prayers whatever you normally do for these daily prayers. The extra prayers and the rituals leading up to them must precisely resemble what you actually do on your own rituals and prayers. The only difference is that you do the extra ones as part of my orders for you. The same is true about the showers. You do your normal daily showers once or twice. And then, you take one or two more showers in line with my orders. The showers must also be completely similar to your real, daily showers. Now, we need to assign certain times during the day when you can do my orders.

At the last part of the session, the therapist, the wife and the husband agree on specific times when the extra prayers and showers can be done.

Session Two

T: It's a pleasure to meet you again. Please tell me what you did.

C: I did what you asked me to do; and sometimes, I couldn't do them. But I didn't get that much better, as I expected I would.

T: Well, what do you mean by that? What happened? What do you mean by no much better?

C: I thought everything would suddenly change. But I still felt distressed at times. I was distraught. When I repeated them one more time, I had the same stress and worry.

T: Last session, you explained to me exactly what had happened. You explained the quality of the problem to me based upon which I gave you some tasks. It's just like visiting a doctor. The doctor prescribes some pills for the patient. The patient takes them and then reports on them to the doctor. The pills gave me headaches, she might say, or, they made me sleepy. They were useless, someone else might answer. You did certain things. Now, I want you to explain to me exactly what you did and what happened.

[6] In this case, that the couple have come to the session together and the husband openly criticizes the wife for her problems, The PTC Therapist tries to change the meaning of the symptoms based on the systemic assumptions of the PTC model. Changing the meaning of the symptoms, or removing the critical attitude toward the symptomatic part of the system, reduces the pressure and the burden on the patient. Meanwhile, the positive attitude of other system members (in this case, the husband) creates alliance and cooperation between the members in solving the problem and makes the relationship between the members (in this case, the relationship between the husband and wife) more dynamic and productive.

C: Well, the home works really tired me, because they were a lot. I really wanted to get better, so I did them whenever I was at home. But I thought that the exercises would make me a lot better, which they didn't.

T: Why did you expect them to suddenly change everything, in the first place?

P: (laughing) Well, they were your prescriptions.

T: I know they were my prescriptions. But why did you expect that? Did anyone say anything to you?

C: No, but others who knew I'd seen a psychologist for my problem, kept asking "are you a lot better? Have you changed much?".

T: Look, when we go to the doctor for some problems, we mustn't necessarily expect to get better right away. We may have a headache. We take some pills and the headache goes away immediately. But, when the pain is in your back, you can't expect it to be healed with a sedative. The doctor wants you to follow a certain diet, to exercise regularly and so on. In this case, you won't get better in a day or two. You must follow doctor's orders for a long time in order to see some improvements gradually.

C: I said the prayers you prescribed really easily. I had no problems at all. For example, I called my children to come to the table for lunch. I realized that it was time for the prayers you prescribed. I said the prayers and came back by the time my children had come to the table. It took less than 10 min. Still, when I want to say my own prayers, it takes 30 min and I don't feel satisfied when I'm done. I leave the room in a bad mood and everybody realizes what has happened. I can't bring myself to say my own prayers as easily as I say yours. I even called a religious reference. I have called him so much that he has gotten to know me really well. He said to me "you doubt too much. If it happens again, saying prayers will be Haram[7] to you." He explains it all to me, but I simply can't get it in here (pointing to her head).

T: You said something that can be a good criterion. You said that you can say the extra prayers easily, rapidly and without any stress, but the real prayers always came with stress and difficulty.

C: Yes, yes.

T: Now, let me ask you this: is the stress you felt during the last two weeks higher or lower than the stress you felt before?

C: Sometimes, it was just as severe. But at other times, I was able to say the prayers fast enough and I felt satisfied after two times.

T: Through the last two weeks, how many prayers were like before, and how many of them were less stressful? Can you tell me in percentage terms?

C: I guess I was better than before, in general. I don't know, maybe I expect too much of myself.

T: We will talk about whether you should have such an expectation or not as we move on. So, you said my prayers easily, and you were able to say some of your own daily prayers with ease. Give me a percentage.

C: For example, we had guests once within the last two weeks. I was able to say the evening prayers easily, but the night prayers were very difficult. I repeated them 6–7 times, and I was really anxious. That is why I can't give you a specific percentage.

T: Just make an educated guess. The wife asks the husband to give a percentage.

H: I think it's somewhere between 10 and 20%.

T: And what about the showers?

C: I took the showers as before. Formerly, I just took showers in the morning. But then, I had to take another one in the afternoon.

T: So you took showers twice a day?

C: Yes, twice. No, it was three times, actually. But I didn't do the last time, sometimes. Sometimes, I couldn't do the last shower.

T: Well, you mentioned the difference between two types of prayers. What about the showers?

C: It was the same with showers, as well.

H: The doctor is asking whether the extra shower was different from the original one or not.

C: Since I knew I was to take another shower, I didn't change my clothes. Because normally, I changed my clothes after each shower.

[7] Religiously forbidden.

T: But they were similar in terms of length, the number of Ghusls and the levels of stress, right?

C: More or less.

T: I need a precise estimation, an exact report on what happened.[8]

C: Maybe it was a little better.

T: Look, you can't expect to get rid of the problem you've been dealing with for six years in an instant. It's not right. No one must ask you about the process of your treatment, and you must not behave in such a way as to let them ask you. You've been having a problem for six years. You can't be treated in two weeks. I would like it to happen, and so would you. But is it a realistic demand? No. You are not even taking medication so that we can expect the chemical effects of the medication to create immediate changes; such as sleeping pills that help you sleep. Here, you want create changes for yourself with behavioral exercises. The reason I insist that you give me a percentage is that I want you to draw your attention to the amount of change you've been able to make. Otherwise, I know you may not be able to give me a precise number, and I don't need such a number in the first place. We do all this to draw your attention toward the change. What is important here is making change, and maintaining the change already made. How big or small that change is doesn't matter to us right now. Our ultimate goal is to treat you completely. But when this goal might be achieved is not definite. We need to be patient and follow the orders for attaining that goal. If there is enduring change, it means that we are on the right track. Now, according to your reports, there have been changes up to 10–20% in some cases. In such cases, you've been able to say your own prayers with your mind relatively at peace. It means that we have found the right track. We have been able to decrease the pressure a little. Now, we need to continue along the same track in order to attain our ultimate goal.

I also need to add that our plan is a short-term one. It won't last long. But even a short-term plan must be within reason. You should consider a three-month period for your treatment. I think treatment within three months is reasonable for a condition that has been with you for six years. We schedule our next session for the next week. In the following week, do the tasks I gave you in the first session.

H: Doctor! I keep telling her that she must want to get better and must help herself.

T: (to the wife) What does your husband mean by saying that you must want it yourself?

C: He means that I have unconsciously convinced myself that I won't make it this time, either. Therefore, I must try to help myself, and really want to get better.

T: If I've understood you correctly, which I think I have, I must disagree with you on this point. The nature of your problem is in a way that is quite unrelated to will and personal determination. It is not related, because if it was, the person suffering from such a condition would not have waited for it to torture her for six years. It is not up to you, or a religious reference, or your husband, or even me to try to decrease it. Quite the reverse, every time you have tried to decrease it, it has gotten worse. And if you try to do so from now on, it will keep getting worse. As I told you at the previous session, this problem has nothing to do with wanting or not wanting, or with knowing or not knowing. It is all about being able to, or not being able to. I'm trying to help you to be able to do it. Therefore, try not to decrease anything in any way. If your symptoms get worse in any way, that's all right. You still

[8] The PTC Therapist must determine therapeutic tasks or home works for the patient at the end of each session. For this reason, from the second session on he/she must ask the patient to present a detailed and complete report on how he/she has done the tasks and the probable consequences of them. The patient needs to be guided to complete his/her report. Such a report, which is a sort of behavioral analysis, tells the therapist whether the patient has understood and carried out his/her home works properly or not. If not, what has the reason been? This helps the therapist change, correct and improve the way he/she explains the tasks. In case the patient has understood or carried out anything wrong, behavior analysis helps him/her understand his/her mistake and correct it. Behavior analysis also draws the attention of the therapist-patient pair to therapeutic changes. The changes, no matter how small they are, are appreciated, encouraged and interpreted as the right adopted strategy for treatment.

shouldn't try to fight them. It's okay if it gets worse and increases. I haven't given orders for it to be decreased, and you mustn't try to decrease it either. And, it's okay for it to increase. Whenever you think it's worsening or increasing, that's okay. Just let it go.

Session Three

T: It's nice to see you again. It's been a week since our last session. Please tell me what you did.

C: It was the same as before. However, I think that I can say my prayers more easily than before. It was better this week. But, I prefer to not have any stress, which I still do. When I say prayers, I still have the stress, although had control over my nerves. My husband has also realized that I've gotten better.

T: How many times do you repeat them?

C: Because I can say my prayers fluently, I'm much better. Although, I do repeat them sometimes.

T: How many times?

C: Two times, at the maximum.

T: I'm talking about your actual daily prayers.

C: Yes, I mean them. I have no problems at all with your prayers (they all laugh). I say your prayers in five minutes. I can say my evening prayers really easily. But I can't say my night prayers. I still have problems with them.

T: What about the noon and the afternoon prayers?

C: I'm fine with them, but I have slight problems with the afternoon prayers as well. My main difficulty is with the night prayers.

T: Now, let me ask one more time, just to make sure. How many times did you say you repeated the main prayers?

C: If I'm not satisfied the first time, I say them two more times at the maximum. I did them up to 15 times, before.

T: And how many times is it for the night prayers?

C: I am talking about the night prayers.

T: What about the evening prayers?

C: I do it just once, unless I think that I might have forgotten something. But it's fine.

T: What do you think is the difference between the evening and the night prayers? Is it the length of the prayers? Or do you worry that you may not be able to do it?

C: It's the worry. I start worrying whether I'll be able to do the night prayers hours before. But I like saying the noon and the afternoon prayers. We were in a party yesterday. It was so crowded, but I just went to an empty room and said my prayers easily. But I still have problems with my night prayers.

T: What about the morning prayers?

C: It's really easy for me. I say my morning prayers only once, and I have no doubts about it at all.

T: What about the showers?

C: That's better as well. Much better!

T: How many times did you do it? Twice or three times a day?

C: Mainly two times, but on two days, I took three showers.

T: What do you mean when you say it is better?

C: I mean I don't fuss over it and don't repeat it. I do two or three Ghusls at the maximum. I just don't know why I still have difficulty with the night prayers.

T: Last session, I emphasized that you must not do anything about your problems on your own. I said that you must simply accept that you repeat them 10 times. The more the better, don't try to decrease them, I said. You left the session with this instruction. Now, I want to put it another way. Last session, I told you not to start saying your prayers with the intention of pressuring yourself to not repeat it ten times. I'll say my prayers once and for all. Or, at least I'll try to make it 9 times, instead of 10. You did as I told you, and I thank you for that. Now, you do Wudu and Ghusl two or three times, instead of ten times. Your new task is to keep it at that level. Even if it was to become less than two or three time, you mustn't let it. You must do them two or three times for some time (*the second complement*). Your previous task was to not try to decrease anything, but it was okay if they decreased for themselves. Your new task is to not let it decrease any more than two or three times. Try to keep it at two or three times, because less than that is not good for you at present (certain justifying explanations—by analogy with the process of losing weight and the necessity of decreasing the pace of weight loss due to health issues—were given here in line with the second complement).

Did you say my prayers during the week?

C: Yes.

T: You don't need to say my prayers anymore. Continue doing the rest of your tasks according to the new orders.

Session Four

T: It's nice to see you again. Please, tell me what you did.

C: Everything's fine as for my prayers. But I still have stress, which disturbs me. My husband says that I'm fine. I say my prayers well enough, but I like to get better.

T: (addressing the husband) What do you think?

H: Now, the only problem is the night prayer.

C: The night prayer really bothers me.

T: How many times do you do it, now?

C: About two to three times. I usually finish it the third time.

T: That's the way it was the previous session and your order was to keep it at that number. This is good. I thought you had gone back to 10 times when you said it bothered you. If it is still on two to three times, it's okay. Because my task for you was to actually keep it at two to three times and to not allow it to decrease. You mentioned something about stress. You talked about it last session as well. Please, tell me about it.

C: We were at a really crowded party yesterday. I was able to say my noon and afternoon prayers easily. But I was so stressed out before that.

T: What do you mean "before that?".

C: I was under stress, because I feared I may not be able to do it right.

T: Do you feel that way in your own home, too?

C: Yes, I feel the same way at home. I like the noon and the afternoon prayers. I can't wait to say my prayers at those occasions. But the anticipation for the night prayer really stresses me out. I get worried over whether I'll be able to do it right or not.

T: Stress over whether you'll be able to say the prayer or not, or whether you'll be able to do it just once?

C: Whether I can do it or not.

H: Excuse me. She means that she is stressed because she wonders whether she'll be able to say her prayers the way she did in the past or not.

C: No, the doctor said that I'm allowed to repeat my prayers and it will be okay.

T: That can be anybody's wish, and that's okay. But it's important to me to hear what she has to say. Because we agreed that she must not try to decrease anything. I want to know what this stress is for. I want to know your own opinion.

C: I get stressed because I wonder whether I'll be able to do it at all, or how much I will be disturbed.

T: All right. We will think about that stress. What else? How were the showers?

C: They are fine. By the way! We are taking a trip to Mashhad on New Year holidays. I keep thinking about going to the shrine and saying prayers there. I keep asking myself whether I can do it in such a crowded place.

T" Look! The problem is now limited to the night prayers. You are now in a period when you need special care so that your treatment would be complete. It's just like someone whose hand has been broken and in plaster. Even when she takes off the plaster, the doctor asks her to not pick heavy things up with it for a month. Because it might be broken again. The patient must be careful and take care of her hand for a while. This trip cannot be good for you at this point. If you can postpone it to some later time, so much the better. But if you have already planned and you must go, you have no other choice. You will probably face no problems on your trip with the plan I make for you today.

Well, after this session, we will have no more sessions for a month, due to the New Year holidays. If you do the task I'm going to give you properly, you will have no difficulty on your trip. Your task about the night prayers is that you must do it three times. Now, let's get to the tasks about that stress.

Starting tomorrow, you must do some mental exercises. Every day, you sit at a quiet place alone for 5 min and recreate for yourself all the stress and pressure you always feel with respect to saying prayers. Re-experience them and feel them just like when they come alive in you and start disturbing you. Try to feel the agitation, worry and stress. Do it twice a day, each time for 5 min (The patient agrees to do one of them 30 min before the noon prayers and the other one 30 min before the evening prayers). Do this for 5 days. From day 6 to day 10, do it only once a day, 3 min before the evening prayers. Then there is the New Year holidays, and I will see you again after the holidays. You must recreate the thoughts about prayers exactly similar to the actual worries and stresses. You may succeed by 100%, or by 50%. Or, you may try and try, but totally fail. Whatever happens, it's fine, as long as you give it your best effort. If you forget to do the exercise in one occasion, it's okay. You simply wait for the next turn to do that. You must not try to make up for the lost session by doing it at some other time.

After the holidays, the patient informed the therapist, through a phone call, that she feels she has been treated and needs no more sessions.

6.3 Assessment of Treatment Outcome and Follow-Up

The course of the treatment was completed in 4 sessions. Assessment of the treatment outcome, which was based on the patients' comments in a graded scale of 0–100 and an open-ended question, indicated 90% recovery. A 2-year follow-up evaluation indicated that there was no relapse.

Client #5 (Male, 15 Years Old, Single) 7

7.1 Case Introduction

SA, a 15-year-old boy, came to the University of Tehran Clinic with his mother. The clinical interview based on DSM-5 (APA 2013) with the patient and his mother confirmed the existence of a series of symptoms related to obsessive–compulsive disorder including obsessive thoughts and doubts, constant washing, orderliness, rituals for going to the bathroom, rituals for taking baths, and constantly checking the lamps and other electronic devices. The disorder which started two years ago, had low intensity at the beginning, but gradually became more severe. It turned into a worrying concern for the patient's family about a year ago. SA has no background of other physical illnesses or psychological disorders, has not taken any medication and does not take drugs at present. This is his first visit to receive professional help. SA was seen for 3 sessions over a period of 4 weeks.

7.2 Course of Treatment

Session One

Therapist (T): (After greetings and the social stage of the interview) tell me a little about what brings you here today.

Client (C): I have an obsession with going to the toilet, saying my prayers and a couple of other important issues.

T: What exactly happens in the toilet?

C: I perform and count a series of actions sequentially. First, I wash my back while counting then I wash my waist and at last I wash the front part of my body.

T: What is the counting for?

C: To keep track of time; for example, I say one, two, three and so forth….

T: How many do you count for each part?

C: I count up to 10 for each part; sometimes it reaches 30.

T: So, the order of washing is like this: first you wash your back, then your waist and at last your front part and you wash each part at least up to 10 and sometimes 30.

C: But there is more.

T: Go on!

C: Each part is divided into some pieces. For example, washing my back is divided into three parts; right, left and middle.

T: And you count to 10 for each part?

C: 10 or more.

T: And do they make it longer for you to go the toilet?

C: Yes. And if my hand shivers, I'll wash it again.

T: You mean your hand should not shiver and if it does, you have to wash it one more time, right?

C: Yes.

T: So, let's imagine you are done with washing, what do you do then? Do you get out?

C: Yes I do.

M. A. Besharat, *Paradoxical Psychotherapy: A Practitioner's Guide*,
University of Tehran Science and Humanities Series,
https://doi.org/10.1007/978-3-031-27717-7_7

T: Do you feel comfortable when you get out?

C: Yes. Sometimes I hesitate but I can solve it on my own by thinking about it.

T: Is there anything else you do before going to the toilet and before washing yourself?

C: I wash my hands beforehand; we have a cat in our yard, and I play with it from time to time and before doing so, I wash my hands.

T: Is there anything you do before washing yourself in the toilet?

C: I roll up my trousers legs so they don't get wet; I wash my thighs after I'm done with the toilet.

T: Do you wash your thighs?

C: After I wash the front part of my body, I wash my thighs to be certain about the cleanness.

T: How many times a day do you go to the toilet?

C: Two or three times; twice if I sleep early, and three times if I sleep late at night.

T: How much does it take you to go to the toilet?

C: Almost 30 min, and sometimes it reaches up to 50 min.

T: You said you have an obsession about saying your prayers; tell me about it.

C: Saying my prayers is getting better because I try not to listen to my thoughts anymore and try to keep on saying my prayers.

T: What did you use to do when you listened to your thoughts?

C: I used to repeat the prayers several times and count them on my fingers.

T: You used to repeat them and count them on your fingers, but you don't have any problems with that now?

C: Now, I say my prayers in congregation and I'm ok. In the beginning, I used to repeat them but I no longer listen to my thoughts and I have no problems with that right now.

T: You said you have an obsession with important issues. What do you mean?

C: For instance, when we are about to leave the house, I tell myself several times that the lights are off, the lights are off, the lights are off; that way I feel sure that they are off; but this is getting better too.

T: Where did you do that? Inside or outside the house?

C: Inside the house. I used to look at the lamp and say "it is off" several times.

T: Were there any problems when you were gone?

C: Not anymore.

T: Did you do it for other stuff too?

C: Electric devices.

T: Did you want to check whether they were off?

C: Yes, but this is getting better too.

T: If we can call these actions compulsive, when did these compulsions start?

C: Before the age of religious responsibility. I was quite sensitive about going to the toilet before but they started last year at the beginning of the age of my religious responsibility (i.e., 14).

T: How does it show itself in performing Wudu[1]?

C: I count the Wudu too; I wash each part twice but it is getting better too.

T: So, you are telling me they are all getting better, aren't they?

C: But the problem about toilet still exists.

T: How about when you are taking a bath?

C: When I think I'm dirty, like when I'm at school and feel like I need to go to the toilet, I go home and take a bath and wash those parts which I think are dirty.

T: How often do you go to the bathroom?

C: Normally or obsessively?

T: Tell me about both.

C: I used to take a bath once a week.

T: What about the last month?

C: It's getting more and more. First it was every other week, then it became every day.

T: How many times have you taken a bath since last week?

C: Last night I took a bath because of a wet dream.

T: How much does it take you to take a bath?

C: Generally, it doesn't take me long; but if I take a bath for an obsession, it will take quite a while.

[1] In Islamic law, *Wudu* is a ritual which involves washing certain parts of the body before one says his/her prayers.

T: So, you have two types of baths: Normal and compulsive. How long does each type take?

C: The normal bath takes 20–30 min and the compulsive one takes 60–75 min.

T: Now, which of these behaviors have become problematic? Because you said some of them have become better.

C: Going to the bathroom and checking the lamps and the electric devices. Oh! When I caress the cat in our yard, I clean my nails with a soap but I don't think it's an obsession. I suppose it's necessary.

T: When you do these things at home, how do other family members react?

C: My mom sometimes gets mad; my father warns me that I might get sick. They are all uncomfortable.

T: What about you? Are you okay with this condition?

C: No I'm not.

T: It's a difficult situation.

C: I'm not okay with going to the bathroom but I'm cool with the rest.

T: Which of the family members are you more comfortable with?

C: I feel comfortable with my mom (I also feel comfortable with my sister, my younger brother and my father).

T: Which of the family members warns you more than the others?

C: My mom. By the way, I don't trust myself either. For example, I take off my underwear to see if it is dirty. Then I take it to my mom and ask her several times to make sure; also, I ask my friends about the schedule many times at school.

T: Do you check them?

C: Excessively.

T: You check the schedule at school and the clothes at home.

C: I ask several times and then I hesitate and ask again and again.

T: Will you be okay if I ask your mom to come to the session?

C: What are you going to ask her?

T: I'd like her to talk about these behaviors and her cooperation. We need her help in the treatment process. Please ask your mom to come in with you.

(Mother enters the therapy session) I heard the general account of your son's problem. I'd like you to briefly tell me about the problem so that I can make plans for the treatment later on.

Mom: SA is very meticulous both about his lessons and his cleaning; he is overly fastidious about anything you might imagine; if he is not convinced, he won't give up. I think this personality trait along with his dependency on me, his father and others have led to these problems.

T: Let's see if SA agrees that he has this personality trait.

C: I used to be like that, but now it's not that bad anymore.

Mom: His problems in going to the toilet have increased for the last few months. He is very diligent and scrupulous in his studies and insists on reaching the goals he has set himself, which makes him even more stressed out.

C: The problem exists both in my studies and in the religious rituals.

Mom: Yes. He usually asks me, and not his father and brother, about these issues.

T: What does he ask?

Mom: The questions are usually about how to perform the ablution.

T: The issues are usually about puberty, taharat,[2] nejasat,[3] and cleaning,[4] aren't they?

Mom: Yes, and he asks so much about them.

C: The questions are about religious issues. They are not about cleanliness and stuff like that. These are religious issues.

T: Yes, they are about religious issues; but all of them, whether the ones you ask about at school or those you check with your mother, have one feature in common, and that is having doubts and hesitations. As you have said before, you ask about these issues to reassure yourself.

C: I have doubts and hesitations.

T: Good! You should acknowledge this to help facilitate the treatment. Saying that the questions

[2] In Islamic law, *taharat* is a general title for several rituals which result in being religiously clean.

[3] In Islamic law, *nejasat* refers to things or persons regarded as religiously unclean.

[4] In Islamic law, things or persons may be unclean and still not be considered as Najis.

are about religious, scientific, and social issues or labeling them as family issues may divert your thoughts from the main problem and prevent you from solving it. All of them have one thing in common: doubts and hesitations. You ask so many questions to reassure yourself; you even said that you don't trust your own eyes; here again, the common factor is hesitation. You don't have an eye problem. You see the same thing even if you look at it 100 times, but your doubts come along and make you check again and again.

Now I'd like to illustrate some points here and I want you both to listen carefully. You need to learn these points. Then, I'll make a treatment plan which you should stick to if you want the problem to be solved. What happens to you (client) is beyond your volition and control. I want you both to pay close attention. If SA washes himself ten times, that's because he can't do that 9 times. If he could, he would certainly do that. If he was able to wash himself 8 times, he would do so. And if he was able to wash himself just once, like others, he would do so and wouldn't do it twice. Here, we are faced with a behavior over which the individual has no control. The person who exhibits this behavior suffers from it more than others and wants more than others to get rid of it, but he can't; because this behavior is not under his control. So SA wants to behave like others but he can't. We'd like SA to behave like others. The problem that SA is facing is similar to that of a person who catches a cold and coughs. The coughing is not under the patient's control and he himself does not like to cough. As we do not blame a patient for his coughing, we should not blame an obsessive person for washing his hands several times, because it is beyond his volition and control. We should not even warn him. Warning is useless here. Warning is given to someone who is able to do the task. We should just help each other solve this problem. When the problem is solved, SA can behave like others and only then will he be able to manage and control his behaviors like others. To solve this problem, I'll make a treatment plan according to which some of the tasks should be done by SA alone and some others with your cooperation (mother).

According to the client's study plans, bedtimes and spare times, the following tasks are prescribed: According to my instructions, in the study days, you should go to the toilet three times a day (at 16:00, 19:00, and 22:00) even if you don't need to. You ought to do the same tasks in the same order that you always do. You should do them with a similar order, frequency and length. You should add two extra tasks to your off days (10:00, 14:00, 16:00, 19:00, and 22:00). Your mother is sitting right here listening to me, and she knows that you will start doing these tasks according to my instructions from tomorrow.

You also have a joint task with your mother based on which you allocate two ten-minute occasions in the study days and four ten-minute occasions in the holidays for asking your mother about religious issues and questions about whether your underwear is clean or *najis* and your mother shall answer your questions as usual. The task for you two is to get together in four occasions (at 11:30, 15:30, 17:30, and 21:30). In such occasions, you can do the tasks just like when you go and ask your mother, the only difference being that now you will do them according to my instructions.

Keep in mind that in all these tasks, you don't have to stop doing your everyday routines or do them within these timeframes. You can ask your mother whenever you have questions and you can go to the toilet whenever you feel so. Be yourself all the time and do not restrain yourself. Only, do my instructions on top of them. If you need to ask your mother ten times, go and ask her and don't keep your questions to yourself. Meanwhile, do the tasks according to plan whether you have any questions in that time or not, and go to the toilet whether you feel so or not.

Session Two

T: Welcome. Let's see what you have done with the tasks and what's happened during the last week.

C: I did the tasks for a few days but I felt I didn't need them so I stopped doing them.

T: What happened when you realized you didn't need to continue doing the tasks?

C: After a few days, I realized I was able to get out of the toilet sooner. For this reason, I stopped doing the tasks.

T: How long did it take you to go to the toilet?

C: It took me ten minutes and then I got out.

T: Does it mean that you no longer had to stick to those rituals, orders and keeping count of your washing in the toilet?

C: Now, I can handle it. If I don't want to do them, I won't.

T: What about checking things with your mother?

C: That too. I did the tasks for a few days and then I could come up with no questions to ask her. Not that there were no questions but that there were a few, and when I asked her, I didn't bug her and I was convinced quickly.

T: In previous session, I heard your report on your rituals in taking a bath and its duration. To make a treatment plan for you, I'd like to know how it went during the last two weeks. Have there been any changes in the way you take a bath, or is it like before?

C: I feel that the duration of my bath has decreased and I was able to take a bath and finish it more quickly. But, I think because I went to the toilet more, as you instructed, I felt I was cleaner and my bath did not take long too. My bath gets longer when I feel I'm *najis*. I haven't felt like that during the last two weeks.[5]

T: Thank you so much. I think you have started quite well and you need to keep on following the rules and do the tasks as much as possible to get the best outcomes. If you just abide by the rules and do not let your own interpretations intervene in doing the tasks, you will achieve a much better outcome. These tasks act like medicine. The difference is that you receive the medicine from the drugstore without changing its content. However, the medicine that I prescribe for you contains things I have determined and you have made and taken for yourself. Here the task gets a little bit difficult and your intervention may change the task I have prescribed you. So keep in mind that you should stick to the treatment plan thoroughly.

For the rest of your treatment plan, which will be in the next two weeks, you should follow the tasks that I have prescribed you about going to the toilet twice a day (at 17:00 and 20:00) and checking your questions with your mother within 10 min (at 21:30). See you next session.

Session Three

T: You are very welcome. You (mother) were not present in the second session and SA's account indicated that he had made some progress, so we decided that he can decrease the number of times he performs each task. According to the treatment plan for the second week, SA was about to do a joint ten-minute task with you and two personal tasks by himself. Now, we're in the third session. Let's see what's happened.

Mom: SA's condition is getting so much better. He doesn't ask so many questions like before. It now takes him ten minutes to go to the toilet. Now, everything seems very satisfactory.

T: Let's hear what SA himself thinks about it.

C: I no longer asked questions from my mother because I didn't have any. The time I spend in the toilet is getting shorter, but I keep thinking about it.

T: What do you mean?

C: In the past, I kept thinking about it and it made me wash myself again and again. Now, the thoughts still exist, but I no longer listen to them and I'm able to stop them and get out of the toilet more quickly.

T: There were different areas that you were struggling with. We only investigated two issues: going to the toilet and repeatedly checking everything with your mother. In the second

[5] This phenomenon seems like the "contagion effect" in some psychological/learning processes. However, reducing this phenomenon, especially in the PTC model of treatment, to the "contagion effect" is lake of validity and accuracy for what has happened here. This can be better explained by what is called "ego strength" in PTC. Practical ability of the ego in the process of the PTC treatment (doing the tasks), aims the heart of the anxiety and distress, disintegrates conflictual dynamics, and processes new psychological powers in a new arrangement. Authority of the ego leaves no space for the anxiety and the pathological symptoms of the disorder. This phenomenon is an empirical evidence supporting fundamental changes in one of the basic structures of the personality (i.e., the Ego).

session you reported that two more issues are getting somewhat better. What about other things?

Mom: He just asked me a question and wanted to know the answer. I don't know in what sexual condition he is. I don't know whether or not he should perform *Ghusl*.[6] I'd like you to talk to SA about these issues professionally.

T: I'll illustrate some points to SA about sexual issues (the rest of the session was allocated to talking to the client about this issue). Apart from that, how was everything else?

Mom: I think the improvement was quite well regarding his obsessions.

T: Have the changes been satisfactory in the last four weeks?

M: Yes, sure.

T: For the rest of the treatment process, two possibilities exist. First, you may have no problems doing the daily activities and you will keep on doing great; or if there is anything that may cause a problem, it is insignificant; like now that the remaining problems no longer cause trouble for you. However, if the compulsive behaviors pose problems for you once again, you have to let me know and make an appointment for another session.

7.3 Assessment of Treatment Outcome and Follow-Up

The course of the treatment was completed in 3 sessions. Assessment of the treatment outcome, which was based on the patients' comments in a graded scale of 0–100 and an open-ended question, indicated 85% recovery. A 23-month follow-up evaluation showed no relapse.

[6] In Islamic law, *Ghusl* is a term referring to the full-body purification mandatory before the performance of various rituals and prayers, for any adult Muslim either after having sexual intercourse, having a wet dream, or masturbating with orgasm.

8 Client #6 (Female, 27 Years Old, Married)

8.1 Introduction

Mrs. ZA, who is 27 years old, came to the University of Tehran Clinic because of suffering sexual impulses and conflicts that were, she believed, caused by masturbation. ZA got married three years ago with the expectation that marriage would get her rid of the need to masturbate. But, the expectation was not happened leading to further conflicts and severe religious guilt resulting from her perceived nightly masturbations. ZA's masturbation started at age 5, when she realized it gave her pleasure to press against her sexual organ. Severe religious guilft made her stop doing it 6 years ago (three years before her marriage). However, it reappeared as perceived masturbation that occurred nightly in her sleep. Compulsive behaviors started when she was 14, including constant washing, exaggerated concern about personal hygiene, taking long baths (for 75 min), doubts before and during saying the prayers and checking the gas valve and door locks. The clinical interview based on DSM-5 (APA 2013), confirmed ZA's OCD. ZA visited a psychiatrist when she was 18 and took sedatives for a short period of time. She has no other history of physical illnesses or psychological disorders, and it's been about 10 years she has not taken medication. This is her first visit to receive psychological treatment. ZA was seen for 3 sessions over a period of 4 weeks.

8.2 Course of Treatment

Session One

Therapist (T): (After greetings and the social stage of the interview) What brings you here today?

Client (C): I had difficulty going to the toilet since I was a little girl. Sometimes, I didn't go to the toilet when I felt the need. Little by little I realized I enjoyed it when I pressed against my genital area. Gradually I got used to it, but I didn't know this was a sinful and harmful deed until I entered the middle school and one of the teachers said it was a sin to do so.[1] Then I realized it is also a bad thing to do and about five or six years ago, two years before I got married, I quit doing that.

T. What do you mean by "doing that"[2]?

[1]. In Islamic law, any kind of sexual self stimulation is considered as forbidden masturbation.

[2] The quitting a strong desire which started when she was five years old, is an example of a complete repression which the "Ego" uses against the demands of the "Superego"; a mechanism which although has seemingly satisfied the needs of the Superego but was not able to soothe the Id and as a result the Id insistently lingers on in forms of sexual behavior during sleep. This excessive repression is one of the symptoms of the weakness of the "Ego", which provides the ground for this disorder. Turning this weakness into the "Ego" strength for managing the needs and demands of the Id and the Superego is the main objective of the PTC model of treatment.

M. A. Besharat, *Paradoxical Psychotherapy: A Practitioner's Guide*,
University of Tehran Science and Humanities Series,
https://doi.org/10.1007/978-3-031-27717-7_8

C: It was a kind of masturbation. I thought it would go away by the time I got married and therefore I quit. It's been three years since I got married and I don't need that anymore but it automatically happens at night. Because I can't do it during the day (it's a sin), it's become so weird. This happens when I'm asleep and then when I wake up in the morning, I feel nauseous and dizzy. I get a headache and become quite aggressive.

T: What happens when you're asleep? Do you have dreams or do you do anything?

C: It's not like those kinds of dreams. It happens by me pressing against the genital organ. It doesn't happen through thinking (imagination). It occurs by physical pressure. I don't know if you can see what I'm saying.

T: I need to know more about it. Masturbation falls into different categories (the client interrupts the therapist).

C: I don't have any control over it. After all, I'm married and I don't need to do it anymore. I don't do so during the day. It's been five or six years since I quit that but at night it happens to me unconsciously; the thing is that it has not happened just one or two nights, it takes place every night!

T: What happens every night?

C: I suddenly wake up. Sometimes my heartbeat increases so much that it makes me wake up and then I realize it has just happened. When I have a pounding in my heart and feel the pressure, I realize that it has occurred a few seconds ago.

T: I don't understand the pressure.

C: I do that for sexual satisfaction.

T: Do you press your body with your hand? Or do you press your legs against each other? How do you do it?

C: I don't press it with my hand. I just press my legs against each other.

T: You do so to press against the genital organ, and by that you become sexually satisfied.

C: Yes. I don't think about it any longer but because it's been with me since childhood, it's become a habit for me. I didn't know it was a bad deed. Since that teacher told me this condition is accompanied by heart pounding and pressure, I came to understand what it was. I studied a little bit and found out about its adverse consequences and I don't like it at all. I feel dizzy, my head aches, I get nervous and I feel uncomfortable about it. I didn't know whom I should visit. I went to a gynecologist and she couldn't detect the problem. I know my problem has a psychological basis and is not physical. The gynecologist said the problem would be resolved by getting married. Two years later I got married. The doctor said I would be okay the next year. It's been three years now and I'm not okay yet.

T: Does it happen every night?

C: Yes! Oh God, I'm exhausted.

T: The problem is that you press your legs against each other, you have an orgasm and then you wake up having nausea, and a headache. Is that right?

C: Yes.

T: How is your relationship with your husband going? How is your sexual relationship?

C: When it coincides with this problem (the coincidence with the orgasm during sleep), I have no sexual desire. Because even if I sleep for an hour during the day, this problem happens and because I feel awful and get this headache, I don't like to have intercourse. May I say how often we do it? (T: Yes.) My husband is not willing to do it (sexual relationship) a lot.

T: He is not willing?

C: No he is not. Does it have anything to do with this issue?

T: I'd like to know whether he likes to do it or not?

C: He doesn't like to do it very much. His desire is average; twice a week.

T: Has he always been like this in the last three years?

C: We had more sexual intercourse at the beginning of our marriage; but it's now become twice a week, at most three times a week but no more.

T: So tell me how your sexual relationship is. How long does it last when you both want to have sexual intercourse? How long does it last from the beginning till the end? What about the foreplay and the intercourse?

C: Overall, it takes thirty minutes and the intercourse takes five minutes.

T: Does your husband reach orgasm during this five minutes?

C: Yes.

T: What about you?

C: If I don't have orgasm before the sexual intercourse (i.e., during sleep), I'll reach an orgasm too. At first, it was very difficult for me because I reached an orgasm during sleep and at the time of sexual intercourse, I'd hardly reach an orgasm.

T: When having sex, does your husband have a full erection? Does his penis become hard and stiff?

C: Yes and he tries very hard to help me. He is not the kind of person who only sees himself.

T: You mean he doesn't ignore you. Very well. Do you have pains or any specific problems during sex?

C: No I don't.

T: Do you become sexually aroused, feel pleasure and have orgasm?

C: Yes.

T: Right. Having sex takes place two or three times a week and whenever you reach an orgasm during sleep, you have little desire during sex and if you don't, you have an orgasm during sex. You accidentally found out that when you press your legs against each other, you enjoy it.

C: Yes.

T: And you have enjoyed it ever since you did it six years ago; that is, two years before you got married. Someone told you this is a bad and sinful deed and you stopped doing it.

C: Yes.

T: Later on you got married. Two years before your marriage, you no longer did it during the day. Is that right?

C: Yes.

T: Did it start at nights two years before your marriage? Or did it happen when you got married?

C: It had started two years before I got married. The thing is that when I masturbated during the day, I was sometimes sexually aroused at nights but when I stopped doing that during the day, it only happened at night during sleep.

T: Does it always happen in the same way? That is, pressing the legs against each other?

C: Yes and when the pressure is high, I feel pain in my heart, neck, the back of my head and knees.

T: How long has it been with you?

C: It started from the very beginning. It's been five or six years that I've felt this way and I didn't know which doctor to visit.

T: I'm asking whether it's been the same in all these years. You've been doing this only by pressing your legs against each other. Right?

C: Yes.

T: You've always done that in a resting position by pressing your legs against each other and not for example by touching yourself with your fingers.

C: Not at all.

T: You mean you didn't do what a husband would do to his wife?

C: No.

For the rest of the session, the similarities and differences of sexual pleasure were discussed in different sexual positions and it turned out that the woman felt relaxed only in a traditional position and did not like to be on top at all..

T: You said you've had a little compulsion. What do you mean by compulsion?

C: I had a little compulsion since the third year of middle school, but I felt better later on. The year after that, I totally forgot about it till last year when my compulsions started once again.

T: What did you do when the compulsions started in the third year of middle school?

C: I had compulsions with washing my clothes and when someone touched them, I washed them again. I was only sensitive about my clothes and my body and nothing more.

T: You mean you were obsessed with nejasat and cleaning?

C: Yes. I always have obsessive thoughts. I'm always careful not to annoy my friends. I always forget whether I've not turned off the oven or not. I'm always obsessed. I think I may have forgotten to lock the door. I have obsessions for different things.

T: What do you do with the oven and the door lock then?

C: I go and check them.

T: What else?

C: I take a bath and wash my clothes.

T: How long does it take you to take a bath?

C: An hour, even if I just want to take a shower.

T: Does it take any longer?

C: Sometimes yes.

T: Has it ever taken less?

C: When my husband comes and tells me to stop, I get out of the bath quickly. If someone is next to me when I'm taking a bath or washing my clothes, like my mom or my husband, I stop. I go to the bathroom and wash myself and when I get out, I feel I'm not clean.

T: Did all these start last year?

C: Yes.

T: So all your obsessions revolve around being najes or clean, washing your clothes and checking things.

C: I'm always struggling with myself and I don't enjoy life at all. For instance, I go somewhere to enjoy and this thought comes to my mind that I've not said my prayers completely. I know it's not true but it seems as if a terrible thought always bothers me.

T: Are the thoughts fewer when you are relaxed?

C: Yes. I feel the same when I try to study. For example, I check to see whether I've read correctly or not.

T: If we call these constant checking and washing compulsions, what comes to your mind at the time of these compulsions? You told me you thought you had not said your prayers completely. What else comes to your mind and bothers you? Tell me about unpleasant things you don't like which come to your mind nonetheless.

C: There isn't anything else. There is something though. For example, when something sticks to my body, such as nail polish, I think it cannot be removed. I always feel that part of it is not removed.

T: What have you done so far to solve these problems?

C: For example, I take a bath and ask my husband to come and call me. At the time of saying my prayers, I count with my fingers; I tell my husband to check the oven; and about my compulsion, I count to three. Then it's over. That way, I can get my clothes quickly.

T: So these are what you did to help yourself. Have you consulted a specialist? Have you taken medicine?

C: Before the university entrance exam, I thought I became weak because of this issue (masturbation) and the back of my head burned, I felt pain in my neck and waist and I felt suffocated. I was sad and depressed and I wondered why this was happening only to me. At that time, I visited a psychiatrist but I didn't tell him anything about this issue (masturbation). I told him I was nervous and he prescribed a tranquilizer. I've not visited any doctors for my compulsions and related problems since then.

T: Did you visit the psychiatrist for just a single session?

C: Yes, about the time of university entrance exam.

T: Do you take medicine right now?

C: No I don't. You asked about my doubts. For instance, when I want to take a nap, I think it's happened again (orgasm) and I feel doubtful about whether or not to wash my clothes.

T: Do you feel doubts about whether you've had a wet dream?

C: Yes. I always think my prayers are not religiously acceptable.

T: Aside from the occasion in which you accidentally found out the pleasurable pressing against the genitalia, have you had any other experience? For example, in relationship with someone else?

C: No I haven't.

T: Very well. Based on what you said, I'll make a treatment plan for you which you should stick to (the client interrupts the therapist).

C: Will it possibly end someday?

T: Hopefully yes. Will your husband attend the sessions if necessary?

C: Yes.

Among issues raised during the session was education[3] *about sexual behavior in order to correct erroneous beliefs and fallacies about sexuality, sexual pleasure, and personal satisfaction and its potential effect on feelings of self-blame and guilt. The treatment goals were explained and defined in different domains.*

T: The treatment plans and instructions in the session act as medicine; you need to stick to the plan carefully to get the best outcomes. Regarding the sexual issues, do the self-stimulation on odd days once; force yourself to reach an orgasm and have a wet dream at night. Decide, think, crave, and convince yourself to have an orgasm. You can do this much when you are awake, and later, when you are asleep, you may or may not have an orgasm. Your relationship with your husband should move on like before till you both come to the therapy session and then I'll make a treatment plan for you both.

Regarding your compulsions, your task is to check the oven and door locks twice a day for five minutes just like other times when you do it. No matter what you think about or feel like while checking, just do as I tell you. Anyway, you need to repeat this behavior for five minutes. Now let's agree on two occasions for doing the tasks because you ought to do them only on these two occasions (after consulting and considering the time limits, we decided that 7:00 would be the time for her to do the tasks during the days she had classes, 9:00 for the days she didn't have any classes, and 22:00 for the nights).

T: And about taking a bath, how often do you do it?

C: Once every two or three days. As a matter of fact, when I take a bath every other three or four days, my compulsions decrease but after taking a bath, I become clean and as a result I need to be more careful and then my obsessions increase.

T: What time is more suitable for you to take a bath?

C: Because I may have a wet dream at night, I usually take a bath during the day and for that reason, I don't do that at night.

T: If you happen to take a bath during the day, what time do you prefer to do so?

C: I prefer 19:00 because this way I'll be able to take a shower even during the day when I get home late because of my class.

T: How long does it take you to take a bath on average?

C: 75 min.

T: Very well. Tell your husband that I have demanded that you take a bath at 19:00 and you are allowed to stay in bathroom for 75 min. Whatever happens, he should not either meddle in or say anything about it; I mean it shouldn't be like before when your husband occasionally came and asked you to get out of the bath. Don't do that anymore. Your mother cannot intervene either.

C: Can I take a bath at morning on days when I'm home?

T: If you would like to take baths five times a day for whatever reasons, you can do so. But for the next two weeks you should take the 19:00 bath just as I have instructed you to do.

Session Two

T: (The patient attends the therapy session with her husband.) It is nice to meet you. (addressing the husband) I had a session with your wife and asked her to bring you so we can get help from you for solving the problem. I'd like you to explain the problem in your own words.

The husband explained the problems just like his wife in her first session. They have been married for three years and have no children. The man is self-employed and his wife is currently a student. The man is not aware of the effect of the woman's problem on their marital life and is not curious to know about it either. Meanwhile, sexual education was offered in this session and the woman's erroneous beliefs about sexual issues were challenged in front of her husband.

T: Last session, I made some treatment plans for you (woman) which you were supposed to

[3] Education is by no means a part of the PTC treatment. Here we are talking about sexual issues and, as is the case in sex therapy, sexual education becomes essential because educational and cultural issues are a necessity here.

share with your husband and follow. Please tell me what you did and what happened.

C: My compulsions about taking a bath decreased a little bit; and about checking, when I close the doors, I feel certain that I've done so. And because I had no tasks on washing, I've been the same in that respect.

T: You said your compulsions about taking a bath decreased. What do you mean?

C: Because I took a bath every day, I was no longer sensitive about it.

T: How long did the bath take?

C: Thirty minutes.

T: You were allowed to stay in bathroom for 75 min; your bath ended in 30 min. So, can we say the duration of your bath decreased in comparison to the past?

C: Yes.

T: And when you get out of the bath, you become less sensitive about touching things, right?

C: Yes.

T: I asked you to check the oven twice a day for five minutes each time. You said that you did. Did you check the oven on any other occasions?

C: If I wanted to go somewhere, I did; but I no longer thought about it.

T: Is there anything different compared to the past?

C: It wasn't obsessing my mind anymore. I sometimes felt doubtful about whether I had done the tasks or not, and then I remembered that I had.

T: Were there times when you remembered not doing the tasks?

C: No there weren't.

T: So you always remembered that you had done the tasks and felt more comfortable in this respect. (C: Yes I did) What else did I ask you to do?

C: During the first week, I masturbated three times but I felt reluctant to do it.

T: What happened at nights?

C: There were no changes at night. They may have decreased a little bit but they were still the same.

T: So you said you dreamt every night and woke up realizing that you had a wet dream and… how many nights within the last two weeks did you felt that way?

C: I can't exactly say whether it happened or not, but I can tell it must have happened because of my fatigue.

T: How much have you suffered from fatigue during the last two weeks?

C: I felt exhausted and reluctant two or three times but it was not severe.

T: So, we have passed 14 days. In the past, you thought based on evidence that the same experience happened every night. Right?

C: Yes.

T: During the last 14 days, you said you found those evidences (exhaustion and reluctance) just in two or three days. Right?

C: Yes. Two or three times.

T: As I instructed, you did the tasks on three occasions on odd days, but for the rest of the odd days (the second week), you didn't do that because you didn't like to. Were there any difference between the first and the second week?

C: No. I didn't feel any differences but generally my sexual desire improved.

Certain questions were asked about the quality of their sexual relationship and some plans were made regarding their relationship to prepare and activate the couple for a richer marital life after the woman's problems should solve.

Regarding your (woman's) personal treatment plan, you need to do the personal sexual behavior (masturbation) twice a week on Sundays and Tuesdays. Continue to take a bath according to the previous plan. Do it once a day at 19:00 with a permitted duration of 75 min. And do the checking every other day just like before. Do this task on even days. For the rest of the obsessions, just focus on your doubts for the time being. Repeat the doubts and hesitations for five minutes twice a day on odd days according to the same plan you had for the previous tasks. Repeat the same doubts about whether or not to wash the clothes (doubts about washing yourself and your clothes); or repeat any other doubts that you may have in your mind.

Session Three

T: You are very welcome. Last session I asked you to do a couple of tasks, please tell me what you have done.

C: I did some tasks about my doubts and thoughts but there were nothing more. I think it is better to postpone it to holidays. I did the checking task but I no longer think about these issues.

T: So you did it several times and then there was nothing left. You believe it's related to the exams. This is not important. What is happening right now is that those doubts and hesitations do not exist anymore. If they happen to come again, we will work on them and if they don't, it will be okay. You said last session that the checking decreased, right?

C: Yes. I've quit doing them. Checking's are not exist anymore.

T: We had two tasks on sexual issues. One task was about your husband and the other was personal. Right?

C: I did the personal task. You said I should do the tasks twice a week but this time I did them willingly and if you hadn't instructed me otherwise, I could've done it every day; I don't know why I was like that.

T: I told you to do the personal sexual behavior on Sundays and Tuesdays. You said you did it on those two days and liked to do it even more. (C: Yes) while you did not like to do it at all in the past (C: Yes), is that right? (C: Yes). You didn't like it and got annoyed but know you've done it in these two tasks and felt comfortable and you were even willing to do more. Weren't you?

C: Yes. In one week, I did it three times instead of two.

T: Very good! This progress is remarkable! How was everything with your husband?

C: Report on the progress of marital relationship was explained.

T: How was everything at nights during the last two weeks? Was that experience repeated? If yes, what were its effects?

C: It wasn't much at times when it happened. I didn't have headaches, nausea and fatigue. I've got better.

T: How is your bath?

C: Taking a bath has become better. Usually it takes 15 to 20 min. I don't like to stay in the bath for long.

T: Very well. Under the current circumstances, your compulsions with checking things, taking a bath and sexual issues and their dire consequences are resolved and are over and done. The rest of your problems about washing, clothes and marital relationship can be solved in one or two more sessions. Since you are having exams, just continue your tasks with your husband on sexual behavior and keep on doing the personal sexual behavior twice a week. When your exams are over, you can continue the session after the summer holidays. Good luck!

The couple re-visited to continue their therapy after 11 months.

8.3 Assessment of Treatment Outcome and Follow-Up

The course of the treatment was completed in 3 sessions. Assessment of the treatment outcome, which was based on the patients' comments in a graded scale of 0–100 and an open-ended question, indicated 100% recovery. A 32-month follow-up evaluation indicated that there was no relapse.

Client #7 (Male, 26 Years Old, Married)

9

9.1 Case Introduction

Mr. ES, a 26-year-old married man, came to the University of Tehran Clinic complaining about panic attacks, fear of driving, and fear of death. He has recently married and is living with her wife with no children. The clinical interview based on DSM-5 (APA 2013), confirmed his panic disorder and agoraphobia. Following panic attacks, ES *feels he is about to die*. Panic attacks and fear of dying make him go to the hospital all the time to receive sedatives. ES is also taking medication because of his gastro esophageal reflux disease. ES comes from a family in which his mother and elder sister both have had serious anxiety disorders for years. However, ES stated that his panic attacks and fears of death started 2 years ago. Becoming more serious, the disorder has badly influenced his job as well as the relationship with his wife. This is ES's first time visiting a clinical center to receive a psychological treatment. ES was seen for 5 sessions over a period of 12 weeks.

9.2 Course of Treatment

Session One

Therapist (T): (After greetings and the social stage of the interview) please, tell me why you are here.

Client (C): My problem started two years ago. I was going on a trip with my family. We were in the car when I suddenly felt sick. My heartbeat increased and I couldn't breathe. It was so bad that I had to get off the car and lie on the ground by the road. My blood pressure dropped, and I thought I was about to die. The same condition happened to me when it was a misty night for the second time. I felt very bad and keep thinking that I didn't have access to any hospitals or something. This fear of not having access to hospitals made me feel worse. Everyone kept saying "you make things worse for yourself and make yourself more afraid." My pressure dropped to 5 or 6, my heartbeat increased insanely and I couldn't breathe. From that time on, I feel some sort of stress or fear of roads. I have to travel between cities due to my job. I was quite the contrary before this. I loved roads and driving. Since 5–6 months ago when this happened to me, I cannot do my job. For about a month, I've been rejecting job opportunities that involve travel. I feel stressful, fearing that it might happen again. I know it's not logical, but it has really affected me. Three weeks ago, I was driving in the city when I suddenly felt the fear. I immediately went to a hospital. When these moods occur, I just want to get to a hospital. I think that if I don't get to a hospital, I may choke to death.

T: Are you afraid you might lose your life whenever you are driving on the road or in the city?

M. A. Besharat, *Paradoxical Psychotherapy: A Practitioner's Guide*,
University of Tehran Science and Humanities Series,
https://doi.org/10.1007/978-3-031-27717-7_9

C: That's exactly how I feel.

T: So, is that what you mean by stress and fear?

C: Yes, fear of death.

T: What else?

C: These problems have really shaken my spirits. I have lost my self-confidence. I always confronted the ups and downs of life and helped everyone around me. Now, it's quite the reverse.

T: I can't understand why it started two years ago. What do you think?

C: I suffered from stress even before that incident, but I was never afraid of roads. Three months ago, this fear intensified so severely that when I reached one of the cities near to my home city, I couldn't go on anymore. I was so close to my home city, but I had to spend the night at my relatives'. I had been feeling stressful from before, but my breathing go heavy all of a sudden, my heart started beating madly and I felt nauseous. I reached the city by midnight one way or another. I stayed there for the night. I took a sedative, went to sleep and took the rest of my trip the next day.

T: I realize you weren't driving when it happened for the first time. What about three months ago? Were you driving then?

C: Yes, I was.

T: Has the bad experience you had on the road two years ago happened every other time you went on a journey?

C: No. There have been times when I went on business trips. I was able to go and come back without any problems. Although the fear was with me all the time and made me come back to the city as immediately as possible. But it has been getting worse gradually. As I said, since a month ago, I have rejected any business trips.

T: So, it gets severe and makes you leave the car only when you travel with your family or some companions. Is that right?

C: Yes, I was with my family in all the cases. I think that was one of the reasons. Because otherwise, I knew I only had myself to rely on to get some place.

T: Do you know at what part of the road (the beginning, the middle or the end) the fear and the worry increase and reach their climax?

C: Mainly in the middle of the road. That's when I feel I am the farthest from the city and if anything happens, it is more difficult to reach a hospital.

T: Is there anything else?

C: That's my main problem, which has made me impatient. I have become so irritable. When I'm driving and I get angry, I drive so fast that it gets dangerous. I feel as if I am no longer holding the steering wheel. I can't help myself, and I step on the gas. I always listened to loud music to feel better. Recently, only high speed can help me feel better. I am scared at the high speed myself, but I can't help it. I'm out of control.

T: Does anyone else in your family suffer from a similar problem?

C: My mother has had it since a long time ago. My sister visited you for her problems which were similar to mine, and she introduced you to me.

T: Have you done anything to solve your problem? Such as taking medication?

C: No, it's the first time I'm doing anything for my problem. I go to the hospital all the time, though, so that I can have sedatives. And I take medication for my gastrointestinal disease.

T: What kind of disease?

C: I suffer from gastro esophageal reflux disease for which I take medication. I sometimes take herbal tranquilizers.

T: Well, I will draw a timetable for you based on what you told me. Is this possible for you to go on a business trip until our next session, which is in two weeks? This fear of traveling, which is an important part of your job, must be cured.

C: Yes I can. It's even necessary, but I've been avoiding them. I was supposed to go on a business trip tomorrow, which I rejected.

T: That's good. One of our treatment objectives is to get rid of this fear of driving on roads. You should arrange for several business trips outside the city starting four days from now. You must do two exercises. First, you must remain, for 5–10 min, in a quiet place without any disturbances and focus. Then, you must do the following imaginary exercise. You must try recreate for yourself all the fears, emotions and worries that disturb you while you are on the road. You must make yourself feel palpitations, the chocking and the impending death. In other words, try to re-experience willingly and intentionally everything that bothers you and makes you suffer. If you manage to recreate the fears exactly, you will get the best outcome. Your main task is to do the exercises on a regular basis, quite similar to taking pills every day. But you may fail to recreate the fears by 100% despite your honest efforts. It's okay if this happens, since you have made your best effort. You may also do your best to recreate the fears and emotions, but you fail completely and the result is not similar to the actual experience at all. Again, this is okay, since you have done your best. Finally, you may forget to do the exercise on time because you forget, you oversleep or you simply don't get a chance since you are somewhere or with somebody. If this happens, the time for doing that exercise is gone and you must not try to make up for it on some other time. You simply wait for the next turn. This is because you must either do the exercise precisely on time, or you must not do it at all. Now, give me two times during the day when you can do the exercise.

C: At 8:00 and 19:00.

T: Start your first exercise tomorrow at 8, according to my instructions. There is one more thing you need to know. You will do the exercises at the two times we have agreed on. It doesn't mean, however, that you must try to avoid or get rid of your fears at other times. No! You don't do, think or decide anything related to your problem at other times. You just do the exercise according to the timetable. You mustn't deal with other times and occasions. We can talk about them the next session.

Here's your second exercise. After the fourth day, when you are supposed to start some road trip, you determine three points before reaching your destination that are equally distant from each other: one quarter; two quarters or the middle; and three quarters. When you reach any of these points, you stop the car and you do the exercise we just discussed for 5 min. Then you continue your trip till you reach the other points.

C: That's too hard.

T: I know the exercise for the first three days will be easier for you to do. If you do them right, you will be more prepared for doing the road trip exercises.

Session Two

T: It is a pleasure to meet you. Tell me what you did.

C: I was able to do the morning exercises more easily. I forgot some of the sessions last week, but I could do the rest successfully.

T: There were two kinds of exercises; one at home, and the other on the road.

C: Yes. I went on two business trips. I did well on one of them, and not so well on the other.

T: What do you mean by doing well and not doing well?

C: On my first trip, I tried to do the exercise at the determined distances and it was really good. I felt like the fears were so irrational and ridiculous. On my second trip, I reached the decision that the fears are so childish.

T: I need to know exactly what happened. You went on two trips. You tried to do the exercises. I told you that you may either succeed or fail. It doesn't matter whether you succeeded or not. What is important is how you felt before going on each trip, during the trip and after having finished your trip. Now, please describe to me your feelings.

C: On the first trip, I was so worried at the beginning of the trip, especially since it was at night time which makes my fears worse. As time went by, I felt better and the fears didn't bother me. On the first trip, I kind of had forgotten about the fears and they didn't bother me. But I still have the worry. It's not over and I still think that I may have problems with travelling.

T: You also did the exercise at other times, when you were not on a trip. What happened then?

C: After doing those exercises, I felt I was able to deal with the stress and the problems more easily. I tried not to magnify every little problem.

T: All right. I think that you have taken the first step with success and you've gotten good results. Before telling you what to do next, I must explain something to you. According to my instructions, you were not supposed to think, do or decide anything other than the exercises themselves. You said that the fears didn't bother you anymore; that's fine. You said that you tried not to magnify your problems. That is not fine. I asked you to forget about yourself for some time. When the problem is resolved, you can do as you like. At the time being, you must not make any efforts to get rid of the problems. Quite the contrary, you must welcome any problem that comes to you. Your willing effort to remove or get rid of the problems may have the opposite result. This is against my prescription. My prescription for you is to recreate your problems at certain times, experience them and deal with them. Continue doing the exercises until the next session.

Session Three

T: Welcome. Tell me what you did.

C: Unfortunately, I wasn't so active and couldn't do the exercises. But I generally felt better. I don't suffer from stress anymore. I don't get angry, and I drive more slowly in the city.

T: What about outside the city?

C: I didn't go on any road trips, actually.

T: Was it your choice, or…?

C: No, the chance didn't show up. I was busy giving exams. It wasn't because of the fear of travelling. It is quite the reverse now. I look for opportunities to go on trips. There was this opportunity to go on a trip, which I had to give up due to my exams. Although, the inter-city project I was working for has finished. I'm much better in general. There is a new problem, however, that keeps bothering me. When I see somebody suffering from a medical condition, I'm worries that I might have that disease as well. This fear was with me before, but it has gotten worse. It's so bad that I avoid sick people. I don't know why! It's not with me all the time, but when it happens, it's really annoying. I know it's so irrational, especially since I worked in a hospital years ago, and I encountered people with various diseases. I had no problems with them then. Now, it's different. Seeing all these diseases really disturbs me. I know it's so childish, but it's bothering me. There is another childish worry I've had recently: I fear that if I go to sleep, I may never wake up again. I've been having this fear for two to three weeks now. I don't know where that came from!

T: You said that you are ready to take road trips, but the chance hasn't shown up yet. This readiness is good. But, keep in mind that you still need the road trip exercises. Whenever the opportunity presents itself in the future, you must do the exercise according to the instructions.

As for negative and disturbing thoughts of sleeping and dying, the diseases or any other worries you may have in the future: you must recreate all of them in 5-min sessions using the instructions I gave you. You are familiar with the process now. You have done it several times, so you do not need any further explanations. Try to recreate and re-experience the worries, disturbances and fears in sessions that last from 5 to 8 min. For the first week, do them twice a day for 5–8 min; and for the second week, do them just once a day. When can you do them?

C: At 8:00 and 22:30.

T: See you next session.

Session Four

T: It's nice to see you again. Please, tell me what you did.

C: I did the exercises as much as I could, and the result was good. My problems have decreased greatly, in general. Before this, I constantly had negative thoughts about diseases and fears. They have completely gone away now and I had no negative thoughts during this time. Last week, though, something happened that made me really upset and scared, and proved to me that I'm still unstable.

T: What was it?

C: I detected blood in my urine. I had a test and it wasn't anything serious. But it worried me for two whole days. It was really disturbing.

T: It wasn't anything important from a medical point of view. But it gave you quite a scare, which was not exactly related to the actual problem, and disturbed you. Am I right?

C: That's right. It really disturbed me. I think that this problem has been with me for a long time. It may have been under the influence of my mother's severe stress. The minute a problem like this comes up, my mind immediately pictures the worst which always ends in death. I am the same in other areas of my life as well. In my job, for instance: whenever a problem presents itself, my mind goes to the worst consequences possible.

T: We will deal with this problem later on. You said that everything was fine when that medical problem showed up and disturbed you greatly. You then explained that, in similar circumstances, you always picture the worst case scenario. This characteristic has been with you for a long time, and might have been overshadowed by your other problems with the road trips and the fear of death. That's probably why you didn't mention it in our first session. Now that those problems have been resolved, this excessive worry over things that are not that worrying in the first place has come to the fore.

What did you do about the thoughts you talked about last session?

C: I did the exercises you told me to, and the thoughts had gone away until that medical problem happened.

T: Did you have any trips?

C: No, there were no trips. And the weather has been really bad.

T: You are now in a good condition, since you are familiar with my work and you have made great progress. I reminded you this, because I want to give you a new task which is way more difficult than the previous ones. It is like a very bitter drug. You must recreate and re-experience for yourself all kinds of medical problems. Imagine that they have happened, not only to you, but to your loved ones as well. Take them to their extreme, and imagine that they have ended in death. Do the same about other aspects of your problem, like worrying too much about your job. For the first week, do them twice a day for 5 min. For the second week, do them only once a day, again for 5 min. When can you do them?

C: At 8:00 and 22:30 for the first week and at 22:30 for the second week.

T: See you next session.

Session Five

T: It's nice to see you again. Tell me what you did.

C: I did the exercises as much as I could. Normally, I feel really good during the day. I no longer suffer from the worries and fears. But whenever a problem comes up, I get really disturbed.

T: How many times have such disturbances happened, and how serious have they been?

C: They happened twice. They weren't as serious as the one before, and they went away soon. The one before lasted for two whole days, but the last two were resolved soon.

T: Did you take any trips?

C: Yes, I went on several trips. I couldn't do the exercises on one of them, because I was travelling with a companion. There was no problem, fortunately. In the other two or three trips, my mind was not occupied with the fears and worries when I was doing the exercises. It was as if I had forgotten about my fears, and I felt fine.

T: Well, to sum up: you did some exercises and tasks. When you did the exercise right, the results were satisfactory. We have the New Year holidays ahead. Now, you know that you must live with the exercises for some time. You have learned the formula for doing the exercises, as well. You know that you at prearranged times during the day, you must recreate worries, negative thoughts, fears and the like so much so that you can overcome them. Due to the habitual stress that has been with you since childhood, you have to accept that incidents that are disturbing and worrying for every one by 20%, might disturb you by 40%. This is a personal characteristic that makes you different from others. You must not expect to behave and live similar to a totally relaxed person. You must simply accept this difference, which is due to your anxiety and irritability. I said this, because acceptance is for you a way toward treatment. Acceptance also teaches you to stop taking drugs for overcoming your personality traits, because they will harm you in the long run.[1] We will have a 40 days interval. You can arrange another session after the holidays if you needed one.

9.3 Assessment of Treatment Outcome and Follow-Up

The course of the treatment was completed in 5 sessions. Assessment of the treatment outcome, which was based on the patients' comments in a graded scale of 0–100 and an open-ended question, indicated 60% recovery. A 34-month follow-up evaluation showed no relapse.

[1] This explanation is not the same as the first complement, which plays an anti-anxiety role. Taking into account the strong biological bases of GAD, especially in cases when other family members have similar biological structures and suffer from GAD (at least two other members of the family including his mother and his sister suffer from severe GAD), the patient must accept his limitations so that he can deal with his anxiety and its consequences more readily.

Client #8 (Female, 55 Years Old, Married)

10

10.1 Case Introduction

Mrs. NA a 55-year-old married woman was referred to the University of Tehran Clinic complaining about severe social anxieties which started about 30 years ago. NA's social anxieties have been always coupled with fears and worries about important people in her life or bad things that may happen in the future. Based on DSM-5 (APA 2013), it was determined that NA had the criteria for social anxiety disorder as well as generalized anxiety disorder. She is living with her husband and their only child. NA's disorders have had a great impact on her field of study, her job, and the relationships with her husband and child. NA does not take medication at present and this is her first visit for psychological treatment. NA was seen for 7 sessions over a period of 16 weeks.

10.2 Course of Treatment

Session One

Therapist (T): (After greetings and the social stage of the interview) Tell me why you are here.

Client (C): I've been suffering for a long time from a series of pressures, anxieties and phobias. I think I've had them since a long time ago, but I didn't visit a specialist because I was younger and stronger, or resistance against visiting a doctor, or maybe it was because I thought I had to visit a psychiatrist and take medication, and I was unwilling to do so because of the possible side effects of the drugs, or maybe it was because of my specialty and my job. Anyway, I didn't do anything about them, and they've started to really bother me. The first time was when I was twenty, and I had an exam or a conference the next day. I don't remember exactly. I suddenly felt a temperature, palpitations, hand trembling and all that. I kept telling myself, it's just an exam, no big deal. If worst comes to worst, you will take it again some other time. But no logic worked. I couldn't convince myself at all. I knew I was being unreasonable. There was no reason why I should feel like that. If I didn't do well, I could make up for it. But it was useless. The logic and the anxiety went two different ways. After that experience, the condition recurred several times. Anytime a stressful situation presented itself, the symptoms emerged. The only difference was that I could predict them. I knew that if is going to be a morning report, my problem comes up. I would definitely feel the anxiety. I knew what kind of a disease I was going to talk about. I had greater knowledge than most of the people in the session, and most of them were below me (I was an intern, and they were in their third or fourth years). I even remember that years later, when I was teaching in the medical faculty, I was invited to some elementary school for something, and I felt the same way in there. They are just a bunch of kids, I kept telling myself! At the beginning, the anxiety is so severe I cannot bear it. Maybe

M. A. Besharat, *Paradoxical Psychotherapy: A Practitioner's Guide*,
University of Tehran Science and Humanities Series,
https://doi.org/10.1007/978-3-031-27717-7_10

this was one of the reasons I specialized in a field which doesn't involve many conferences. I prefer it to be just me and my patient.[1] I don't have a problem with a patient or two. But if there is a group, even if I know they are inferior to me, I have difficulty dealing with them. It is okay to feel like this if you are meeting your professor, for example, and you are worried you might say something incorrect. But it's not okay to feel anxiety in meeting somebody who knows nothing. They will accept anything you say. It doesn't work this way for me, however the anxiety is there as strong as ever. Certain symptoms of the anxiety are always with me. I always have a slight tremor which becomes quite noticeable in anxiety-inducing situations. This is my main problem.

T: Well, in sum, you feel like this whenever you have to stand before a group of people and present something. Is that right?

C: Yes, and sometimes, if I am going to talk about an important issue for an important person, even if it is just that one person, this happens and I feel anxious for the first few minutes.

T: It's clear that you feel uncomfortable and anxious under such circumstances. People with a similar condition can sometimes point out what they are afraid of. Can you also tell? Can you tell me what you are afraid might happen?

C: No, I don't know what might happen. I feel like that if it's something important, or it's with someone important, or there is a group of people, I become anxious.

T: Well, you have told me about the problem, and the long history, and the fact that it has gotten worse recently. Have you done anything about it so far?

C: Before my thesis defense session, I took a Propranolol, which slowed down my heartbeat and made me feel better. I did it once or twice, and nothing else. I was not sure whether I should see a psychiatrist or psychologist.

T: Let me give an answer to this question here and now. I think you have come to the right place and you have been right not to see a psychiatrist before. A psychiatrist, in case he/she is able to make the right diagnosis, intends to alleviate your problem by prescribing medication for you. The problem, however, is not solved. And I don't even talk about the side effects of taking medication for a long time. We will use a different method that will hopefully treat you.

C: There is one more thing. Our psychiatry professors asked us how we felt when we woke up. Happy, neutral or unhappy? I usually belong to the third group. I don't remember having woken up happily, ever. I mean, I have never been really and deeply happy. I always made an effort to think of happy thoughts, telling myself it's going to be a great day, full of health and stuff! There is no reason why you must be unhappy. I keep telling myself such things! The truth is, however, I don't usually feel happy with the things that make others happy. And a lot of things that make other people really sad and crying, has no influence on me. Yes, it does make me upset and sad, but I rarely show how I feel by crying out loud and making a scene. I try, mainly, to accept it. And I believe it's related to how I've been brought up (explanations were given about the influence of family and upbringing on lifestyle and life choices).

T: You talked about mornings. We know that you have never felt happy at morning. Does this mean you are actually unhappy, or that you simply are not happy?

C: No, I wasn't unhappy. I'm usually like this, how you see me now. Why don't you smile, my husband keeps telling me. He asked me this especially at the beginning of our marriage, because he is the exact opposite of me and is always laughing. He wakes up happy every morning. I'm like, what is there to be happy about this early in the morning?

[1] Cognition, logic and reasoning are normal actions of the brain and the intelligence, and function according to each individual's intellectual ability and development. However, the essence of psychological disorders is of a completely different nature. Therefore, reasoning does not influence it. The disorder goes its own way, independently. The brain and the intelligence offer solutions such as choosing a less risky specialty. The PTC model, as a paradoxical treatment, has the same nature of the disorder. This treatment is completely alien with cognitive solutions.

T: You said that it is rooted in your childhood upbringing. Can it be due to anything else?

C: No, I don't know. Sometimes, I think that maybe I have a very sensitive, irritable and unhappy personality. The things that have happened to me in life have contributed to the formation of such characteristics. A lot of people would feel really happy and contented with what I have. But I don't think about them a lot (education, career, good children and a caring husband). They tell me about them, and I'm like they don't matter. They have always been there. But thinking that my husband's serious medical condition might get worse in the future and that our child might suffer as a result, I feel so bad that I wish I had a much simpler life and did not have to deal with this problem. My acquaintances, who are mostly educated people, tell me "don't think like that. Accept what you have and who you are. Accept that these are the circumstances of your life and they are beyond your choice." several nights, I suddenly wake up with this worry in my mind and I go say prayers. The worries haunt my mind so bad that I cannot go back to sleep for several hours. Or if I go to bed late at night, the thoughts and fears of the future, things that may never even happen, keep coming to me and I can't go to sleep for hours.

T: This problem of fears and worries about important people in your life or bad things that may happen in the future and preoccupy your mind for several hours, which we call problem number two—how frequent does it happen?

C: I can say that it has increased gradually.

T: Do you think you would still had such a problem if your husband didn't have this condition?

C: Yes, I had my problem before knowing my husband. So, it can't be related to his health condition.

T: That is correct. You have a background of anxiety that fits any situation. There are two things: anxiety, and those fears and worries of talking of important subjects among a group or for important people. The two problems are related to one another. But we need to distinguish between them as two clinical conditions.

I make a timetable for you that includes several daily exercises you need to do, similar to the drug that you must take on a regular basis every day. As for the first condition, I hope you can manage your days in a way that you would not have to be in an anxiety-inducing situation for the first four days. This way, you can do the exercise on your own for a number of days and then test the result in a real situation. You have had some experience in the past, which you can imagine. Recreate those situations in your mind in a way so that you feel the anxiety, fear and worry attached to the situation anew.

C: You mean I should review them.

T: Review them, but in a way that the consequences are identical to the real situation. You review a specific experience, and it hits you as strongly and bitterly as the original experience. The more this bitterness, anxiety and stress is the better. This is the first stage of your task. You must do this exercise successfully for at least a couple of days before you can be ready to move on to real situations. Suppose a real life situation presents itself on the sixth day, a situation that can normally cause fear and stress for you. In this stage, you must divide your exercises to two from the fourth day. Fifty percent of your exercises must be related to stressful past experience, and the other fifty percent about the future situation you are going to find yourself in two days later. Let's suppose you must give a speech in a conference. The second fifty percent of your imagination must be allocated to the conference. You must imagine that you go to the conference and you feel the stress and anxiety you have felt before in similar situations. Imagine that you feel so stressed that you cannot give your speech anymore. You can't even control it this time. In real situations, you are able to control and manage it after two to three minutes. But during the exercise, imagine that you have failed to control it altogether. A disaster! Pay careful attention that what you must do and imagine is contrary to what you did previously. Before this, you did your best to prevent the anxiety from taking place. According to this method, however, you are not allowed to do so. Quite the contrary, you are trying for the worst case scenario. This is very important. If you have the slightest wish to get rid of the anxiety because you have done the exercises, for example, the anxiety will hit you more severely than ever. Your only duty during the exercises (either imaging past experience or the possible future events) is to make an honest effort to experience what I asked you to; a situation harsher than the real life. But, you may not be able to recreate and review the experiences as intensely as possible. If you can do so, so much the better. Otherwise, any intensity is all right as long as you do your best. You must not try to make any changes to my prescriptions and simply stick to what I have prescribed you to do. Do not try to analyze or interpret it on your own. In cases, you may do the exercise correctly, but you fail to recreate the experiences completely. This is still all right, since you have done your best.

C: What if a real situation does not present itself?

T: In this case, you just continue doing the imaginary exercises about the past. Therefore, you will do the exercise up to the next session. Either you just do the imaginary exercises about past experience or, in case there is going to be a real situation to come, you also focus on the future. Starting from tomorrow up to our next session which will be in two weeks, you must do this exercise twice a day for the first week and once a day for the second week. Each exercise must be about 10 min. Tell me the two times, taking into account that you must be able to do the maximum amount of exercises. Also, you cannot change the time you set and the exercises must be done precisely on time. You will either skip the exercise altogether, or do it exactly on time. If, for any reason, you fail to do any of the exercises on time, you skip it rather than trying to make up for it. Now give me two times.

C: 7:00 and 22:00 for the first week, and 22:00 for the second week.

T: Now, let's get to your fear of bad things happening. You must add an exercise related to this aspect from the second week. In other words, you do one exercise for the first problem and two more exercises for the second problem. For the second week, the instruction is the same as the exercise for the first problem. The only difference is the subject of the exercise. In this exercise, you imagine and recreate fears about the health of your loved ones. You discussed worries about your husband. You may have similar worries about other people and situations that you haven't told me about. However, you yourself know about them.[2] Imagine all of them in the harshest and most intense way possible. During each exercise, you imagine mercilessly that the worst thing has happened to your loved one and you feel your worst as a result. Give me the times for this second exercise (the client changes the times for the first exercise to 21:00, and decides to do the second exercise at 7:00 and 23:00).

T: There is another important point to take into account. Your duty is to do the home works at times we agreed on. This does not mean that you must try to control your condition at other times. You do nothing to control, prevent or manage your two problems. You forget all about them and let them be. Whether they come to you and happen repeatedly or not, you have nothing to do with them. See you in two weeks.

Session Two

T: Welcome! Please tell me what you did.

C: I did the exercises, and I did my best, but I managed to make it like the real experience only by 20%, and in real circumstances when the stress came to me, I didn't feel there was any difference.

T: When did this real circumstance occur?

C: It was exactly two weeks ago.

T: Let's analyze the two conditions separately and see what has happened with respect to each.

[2] An advantage to the PTC model is that the client does not need to explain all the symptoms of the disorder and their details in order for the therapist to be able to prescribe therapeutic exercises. Forgetfulness, lack of time or other personal or cultural reasons may prevent the client to tell everything to the therapist. Telling the client "there may be other things you didn't get a chance to talk about, but you know they are there" make her/ him realize that the therapist's orders include the unsaid stuff as well. In case the unsaid stuff seems to be of importance, the therapist can ask the client to talk about them in the next session. This quality is due to the fact that PTC is not a diagnosis-based method.

One was pure imaginary tasks. What did you do about it? Whether the tasks about social anxiety or the worries about your husband and loved ones.

C: I didn't feel much of a difference in either one.

T: To what extent was it predictable for you? Were you able to predict the circumstances of the real life?

C: I had greater focus during the first week, but then, perhaps I felt that it was useless, so I lost focus and my mind was scattered and I had to try to collect my thoughts. But I did my best in any exercise to do at least 5 min of good exercise.

T: Thank you for this explanation. But I didn't mean that. Suppose there is a conference you have to attend; a real life situation. How did you do?

C: It was so out of the blue. It was not a social situation, but it did cause me stress. The tax inspector came along to check our income and increase our tax. It was an important issue, so it caused enough stress. Or, there was another problem about my daughter's school, which was difficult for me for some reason, so it caused me stress. Maybe I have to add that anything that is a more than normal level of importance to me can cause me stress, whether it is a person, or an important issue, or a specific social situation. The more predictable the situation is, the more difficult and stress-inducing it will be for me. If the situation occurs all of sudden and unexpectedly, I may never feel stressed. It's worst when I know that I am going to have a speech in a certain conference at a certain time next week, or meet a certain person, or talk about an important issue. Recently, the pressure has been so great that I prefer to avoid the situation altogether so as to avoid the stress, even if it means that I have to let go of the benefits that situation might offer me.

T: Were the two situations you talked about unexpected?

C: They were both unexpected and so I didn't feel that bad. If they were pre-planned, I would have felt a lot worse.

T: How about the fears and worries related to your husband?

C: He is abroad at the time being; it's been about a month he is outside the country.

T: Do you mean that the worries exist only when he is present?

C: No, but when you have something before your eyes and it happens to you repeatedly, naturally you feel it more pronouncedly. When I think about a fear for some minutes, a series of unfortunate possible events flood my mind. When a negative thought is triggered, the worst comes to my mind. Suppose the worst has happened, I tell myself. You still will have the power to deal with it. But it doesn't help me feel better at all.

T: So, you were supposed to imagine the worst during the exercises. Were you able to do so?

C: Yes, but they still bothered me more during other times of the day than during the exercises. I couldn't feel the stress and worry during the exercises. Let me give you an example. My mother wanted to go on a trip. I told her "you don't know this driver, and his car isn't good. Don't go!" I tried to convince her not to go, but she had to go for some reasons. The night she was about to leave, a series of disastrous events raided my mind. What if she has an accident, what if, what if … I went over all these thoughts in my mind. Then I told myself that a lot of people travel with cars. The picture of people whose spinal cords were damaged in accidents entered my mind. These images and thoughts are so strong that it's almost as if they exist beyond me. Waves of stress bring a racing heartbeat, tremor and perspiration with them quite of their own accord, and all the reasoning I do fails to have the slightest effect on me. That (the reasoning) cannot make them (negative emotions) go away. I know that they have no rational basis. I don't know this one driver, but I don't know a lot of other drivers as well. Or, though his car is not in the best condition, it is still as good as a lot of other cars out there. But these arguments do not calm me at all. I don't know why.[3]

[3] The PTC model does not deal with cognitive processes directly and does not waste the treatment with processes unrelated to the original foundations of psychological disorders. The main reason is the immediate and deep impact of the PTC model through making changes to the emotional and personality causes of the disorder. Cognitive change is a consequence of the PTC treatment process. The reports of this client—a client with a high education and great cognitive skills—during several

T: They can't calm you, and they won't. It's because they don't have such a determining role in the development of psychological disorders. I told you not to make rational arguments during the exercises. All you have to do is to try to experience disastrous thoughts and negative emotions.

According to the report you have given men, I want you to focus on the second condition: the worries about the loved ones such as your mother, your husband or any other person there is. Just pay attention that, as I told you at the previous session and repeated it now, during the exercises, you must make the attempt to imagine the worst event possible and do not stint. The instruction for doing the exercise is as before. Make the maximum effort to recreate it by 100%. There are other possibilities that might occur, such as forgetting to do the exercise, or failing to reach 100%. At other times during the day, you mustn't make any effort to stop the worries from haunting you. Have nothing to do with other times. We will later talk about whether they should come to you at other times or not.

C: Sometimes, I implicitly blame myself for not being able to stop these thoughts from happening. At other times, I feel like I have disease for which I cannot be held to blame. Is this anything similar to a disease?

T: It is totally out of your control; you cannot decide it's coming and going.

C: Is it hereditary, or acquired, or a combination of both?

T: Usually, a series of causes work together to create such problems.

C: I asked this, since my father suffers from similar fears and worries. My father's mother was also like this, even worse. Some of his grandchildren also suffer from this problem; and some of my aunts too.

T: Yes, they have biological bases, and the family resemblances you mentioned can be due to such bases. But they are not all. There are other factors. The anxiety has a different level in each of the individuals you mentioned. Also, there are other family members who share your biological characteristics, yet do not suffer from a similar problem. For this, and other, reasons, it is totally beyond your control. It's just like the disease you mentioned. The individual is not to blame at all. With this timetable, you can experience changes that increase your power to control such emotions and stressful thoughts.

Our present timetable must remain focused on this condition. As for the other condition, the fears about social situations, people and important issues, it is best if you can keep away from real life situations until we have time to focus on it specifically. So, try to avoid it as much as you can. For two weeks, you need three exercises a day for the first week, and two exercises for the second week. Each exercise has to be 10 min. Tell me the times.

C: 7:30, 14:30 and 22:00 for the first week and 7:30 and 22:00 for the second week. Let me tell you something about my childhood. I remember, when I was about 3 to 4 years old, hearing sounds in my head. It was like a hubbub. I closed my eyes and saw formless things that were really tiny, but they suddenly became insanely gigantic, and it was like they were becoming bigger inside my mind, and the voices were there all the time. I tried to make it go away. I left the room and walked around. They happened every once in a while. Later on, when I got to know diseases and disorders, I tried to find out what that was about. I couldn't find out what it was. They still happen at times. Something along with a vague sound, like the sound of a car moving in a tunnel. Then, it is inflated in a millisecond and becomes huge. I try to change it. I always wanted to know what it was. Do you think it's anything important?

T: These symptoms are not important per se. But when they occur in an individual who has suffers from anxiety and stress, it can be claimed that they are related to the problem. Medical causes can be equally the cause. Since it is not a clear clinical condition, it is considered as a minor symptom. We can still rely on conjecture, mainly. Is it due to fatigue? Is it caused by a combination of fatigue and stress? Is it a defense mechanism, a physical and biological one, not a

sessions confirm this theoretical and experimental claim of the PTC model.

psychological one? There are lots of hypotheses to be examined, but I don't think it's important. You do the exercises till the next session. See you in two weeks.

Session Three

T: It's nice to see you.

C: Thank you. I did the exercises. I lost one or two, though. I did three exercises a day during the second week, too. I feel that some knots and pains have been alleviated. It's like my mind is lighter. Bad thoughts emerge less repeatedly. It's less painful by 20–30%. There were some mild stress-inducing situations, too. And I felt I was able to handle them better than before.

T: This report means that the exercise you've done has been effective to a relatively good degree. We had a mild exercise for both problems in the first session. The real life situation you reported for after that session was not predictable so that you can exercise for it beforehand, but it gave us a general idea. Last session, we put our focus on a specific situation and now your report tells us that it has had the expected outcome, and you have been able to penetrate the wall and had created a crevice in it. You must keep doing it until the wall collapses.

Another valuable point you mentioned was that you focused on the clinical condition, that is to say, the worries about your loved one's health, which is the basis of your anxiety. However, the result you got was not limited to that problem, but extended to your other problem which is your special fears. When you found yourself in a situation that normally arouses those fears, the stress and the fear was felt less strongly. This was predictable, since although we are dealing with two clinical conditions, the anxiety-inducing bases of both are the same. That is why we see progress in both areas.

I gathered these conclusions from your own report, so that you can be aware of the value of the work you've done better, and do the rest of the exercises more determinedly. Also, remember that you are in the middle of all your routine responsibilities and occupations, and we didn't stop any of them in order to create a more favorable clinical atmosphere for you. We did not make even the slightest of changes to your normal life.[4]

I want you to continue doing the same exercises for two more weeks. Three times a day for the first week, and twice a day for the second week. Can you do them at the same times as the previous weeks?

C: Yes, they are fine.

T: See you in two weeks.

Session Four

T: Hello, and nice to see you again. Tell me what you did, please.

C: During the last two weeks, and especially during the second week, I was so busy I couldn't do the exercises completely. But I tried my best.

T: How did you feel?

C: I feel that there are things that have for a long time been occupying a part of me, and now they are gradually losing their weight. Sometimes, I feel light. The hours when I feel free have become more frequent. For our session together, I did not feel any stress. But since an hour ago, the thought of the session have been coming back to me. This happens in quite normal situations, as well. A couple of days ago, I was going somewhere with my daughter. She has this habit of tying her shoelaces not until the last minute. Tie your shoelaces dear, I asked her. We will be there in five minutes. She said it didn't matter and that she would tie them up in four minutes. Why do you keep asking me to tie them now, she asked me. Well, I cannot be like that. I tie my shoelaces fifteen minutes earlier, so that I don't get delayed. It was a routine family meeting, and it would have been okay if we were to wait for her to tie her shoelaces later. But I just cannot be like that. In 99% of the cases, everything must be quite ready beforehand. I can't believe that others never worry it might be late. They are so relaxed while I keep worrying it

[4] One of the advantages of the PTC Model is that it eliminates the anxiety immediately and empowers the client so fast that she or he does not need to make changes to her/his daily, normal life. It was based upon this power to have influence that, as we saw in some cases (e.g., in client #3), the patient stopped 10 years of drug therapy with all her self-confidence.

might be late. I always feel like that, and it's so annoying.

T: That is the main problem.

C: I tried a lot not to be like that, but I just couldn't help it. For example, I was in elementary school, and when I got home, I had to finish my homework before changing out of my school uniform. Now, my daughter leaves her homework for the last minute. Last night, she was doing her homework late into the night, after two days of holidays. I was the exact opposite of her. And I'm still the same. I get home exhausted, but I can't think about resting before I make everything ready for the next day and put everything in order. How bad is this? Even if it is bad, it shouldn't cause so much tension. It causes so much tension for me.

T: Before I tell you what I think, I want you to tell me your opinion on why you were like that. It sounds like you had to act that way. You had to do all the homework for the next day before changing your school uniform. Why? Why should everything be ready and in its right place beforehand?

C: It was partly because my mother pressured me. I was the first child, and my family was in a special social situation. There were lots of social expectations from our family and we had to watch our behavior all the time. And then, the first thing within me was my own religious beliefs. I believed I must make the best use of my time. I shouldn't waste a single minute of my time. I always felt like that and I still do. I feel like I'm in this world for a short time, and I have to do a lot, and no matter how much I do and accomplish, it still wouldn't be enough. I remember I was in the fifth grade. I went to school two years earlier. I was in the fifth grade when I was nine. My average was 19.90, and when I showed it to my mother, she was like "fine but, what about this nineteen?" That's all. She didn't say much. She would comment with a word or two.

T: What did she mean?

C: She didn't see all the twenties I got, and her eyes would immediately go to the nineteen. The next term, my average was 20. It was a really hard competition. There were four, five good students in my class. When I showed her my marks, she said "it's good. But it doesn't count as long as you don't get a 20 for your conduct."

T: Weren't there a mark among them for your conduct?

C: Yes, and I'd gotten twenty for that as well. But what she meant was the morality. In other words, the marks didn't matter. And I felt I was always behind the schedule no matter what I do. If my average is 20, still my conduct might not get a good number. So, I have to try harder. If I say my prayers on time, it doesn't count, since you can't tell whether you've done it with real presence of mind or not. Even if all the religious standards are followed, there is still room for improving it. Well, it's all right that I am the top student in the city, and the province. But what about the whole country? What about the university entrance exam? There is always something missing. She is like that, too. She is a very devout and religious person. She has done a lot of good deeds, but when you tell her so she is like "no, my prayers are questionable, and I'm not sure about my fasts". This is how she thinks. She has to reach a summit she is always finding herself short of. She does not have anxiety at all, however. She is the exact opposite of me in that regard. She is quite relaxed and calm. I have used the same methods, but with different results. Or, maybe it stems from somewhere else. I'm not sure. I really feel disturbed. It all bothers me a lot.

T: Thank you for all the useful explanations, which I was curious to know about. However, you didn't answer my question. Before I ask my question again, I need to ask you a marginal question. I want to know your opinion as a religious person. Should all the religious rituals be completely perfect, or does religion accept it as long as we do our best?

C: Well, religion accepts the least bit of effort on the part of most people.

T: Even insufficient efforts are accepted in religion. I want you to pay attention. Religious upbringing does not have to be so harsh. A mother imposes such harsh measures on her child who already has the tendency toward anxiety. A five year old child is not a one of the disciples to be have to appear faultless in her religious conduct. I just needed you to have this in mind.[5]

Now such a mother, who is an apotheosis of virtue, and who has adopted such a lifestyle, aims to apply it on her child completely. In case the child does not have a tendency for anxiety, she may be able to receive this upbringing in a more healthy way. But the child might have the biological background for anxiety, as you do. She has the tendency to suffer from similar clinical conditions with which you have been inflicted, as you know, since childhood. It has influenced you differently, however, as you have grown and have adopted a greater understanding with further responsibilities. It has been with you since childhood, nevertheless. When a child has the biological characteristics, the harsh discipline and the unreachable standards work as a great fire that keeps the flames of anxiety glowing to the extent that the anxiety no longer needs to be tended to so as to remain active. It functions without any outside triggers, spreads everywhere and tortures the person. We reach the stage when there is no need for a fire to keep the flames of the anxiety alive. In fact, the person is worried and decides to put the fire and the flames out, but they can't be extinguished anymore. They are out of control. The flames of anxiety find their own fuel. The person attempts to splash water on them and put them out, but the water is not strong enough to put out the fire, and the fires of anxiety cannot be put out by water in the first place. Other methods must be sought, which is the purpose of what we do here.

Once, a trigger was necessary to create the fire. Now, there is no need for that. Once, an outer motive was needed, but not anymore. The person has become equipped from within. She provides the fuel for the fire from within herself. The child has become a mother and is doing the same to her child. Interestingly, however, her child does not have a similar tendency, so the triggers don't work on her. She is not made of cinder, so she cannot catch fire. So far, none of your efforts have influenced her. You can say that she is carefree and laid-back. It means that both the tendency and the outer drive must be there together, which was the case about you. The two factors worked together to create the clinical condition you are in now. One of the factors cannot do anything on its own; you and your daughter are great examples to this formula.

I asked you why you behaved that way in childhood, trying to do everything on time and prepare everything beforehand. Our discussions showed that you simply couldn't act otherwise. The reason is the fear of not being able to do it later on. It comes from that anxiety, and it is, and has always been, beyond your control. As time went by, it became even more difficult for you to control it. What we are trying to do here is to equip you with the power to be able to control the anxiety, manage it and overcome it in the end (the therapist offers explanations concerning the influence this condition can have on other family members, such as the husband and the daughter, and the help and contribution they can have to expedite treatment. Since their participation in the treatment process was not possible, details of the discussion have been omitted). Have any real life situations presented themselves so far?

C: There was nothing serious, but there were several mild situations, which I was able to deal with better than before.

T: I want to ask you to add this to the exercises you do. You still have three exercises a day, doing the task about worrying for the loved ones during the first and the last exercise. For the middle exercise, focus on the task I gave you in the first session; that is to say, imagination and recreation of social situations that cause stress and anxiety for you. In case there is going to be real life situation, start from at least 48 h earlier and do the imaginary exercises every four hours. Imagine the situation you are going to be present at and imagine that the worst is happening. Don't

[5] Mentioning marginal issues in the economical, short-term PTC model follows psychotherapeutic purposes, and is not done for fun. The present client has a special personality characteristic that necessitates it for her to receive the PTC model of treatment for personality disorder after having dealt with the anxiety disorder. Therefore, highlighting educational determiners along with biological bases, prepares her for receiving the personality treatment later on. Pay closer attention to subsequent conversations, which are related to this issue.

do anything else. Don't think to yourself "well, hopefully I will do this and that and the speech will go really well and there will be no problems." Do not do this at all. Just think about and recreate a total disaster. Before going to that social situation, bring all the disastrous thoughts to your mind. You are actually going there to experience the worst. You are going there to have the worst thing happen to you, and be sure that it will happen.

C: If there is to be such a situation, the horrible thoughts come to my mind four time an hour, rather than every other four hours.

T: Great point! What you are about to do according to my orders must happen every other four hours. What happens other than that, or at other times, is not up to you. If the thoughts come, you can't avoid them. And if they don't come, it doesn't matter. Stick to the previous instruction. Now, give me your times.

C: Same as before!

T: All right. See you in two weeks.

Session Five

T: It's nice to see you again. Please, give me a report.

C: I tried to do the exercises as much as I could. I missed some of them. I don't feel any improvements. I feel just as much better as the previous session, no more. One or two social situations came up, that were awkward and caused a lot of tension.

T: Tell me about one of them. What was the situation, how did you feel before it, and what were you thinking? What happened there?

C: I tried to go there in the mindset you asked me to. I tried not to tell myself that it will be all right, I will do fine and things will go well. It was like before. Negative thoughts occupied my mind, and stress overcame me. Take this session with you, or my other daily routines. Before I am through with them, they keep coming to my mind. Do it at one thirty, one thirty, one thirty! It gets really annoying. And it's the same with everything. Like, today I have to call this doctor. The thing itself is not important at all. Neither the topic of the discussion, nor the person or anything else about it is important. However, the second I open my eyes in the morning, thoughts about it preoccupy my mind. If it is something important, it gets much worse and takes longer before it's over. In appearance, I am doing daily routines, but my mind is elsewhere, occupied with a certain appointment. When I'm watching TV, my eyes and ears are directed at the TV, but I am not. This is really torturing me. Maybe 20 years ago, the number of things that could occupy my mind were very limited. But they have increased and they are mainly pretty trivial matters. For instance, I have to take my daughter to the basketball class at 5. I've thought about it about 20 times since the morning, although it is nothing worthy of attention.[6]

T: So, any number of tasks or appointments that must be done during the day, turn into a series of annoying thoughts that preoccupy your mind and bother you, regardless of how important they are. Is that right?

C: Yes, and now that I compare myself to 5 years ago, I realize that the number of things that can disturb me have increased, and they are mainly things that I know about beforehand. Like, I have to be here at 13:30, or I have to take my daughter to her class at 17 and so on. If things happen unexpectedly, even if they are very important, they don't cause me any stress and anxiety. It's impossible for me to be able to postpone an appointment. I'm ready in my car to take my child to her class. I'm the one reminding her to hurry up. The exercises have been useful in general, but maybe I've been expecting more from them.

T: This expectation is not necessarily bad, and can encourage you to keep doing the exercises. And the slow rhythm of progress is positive, since it helps to make the changes and the improvements permanent. Well, your personal

[6] The patient reports on recurring, annoying thoughts for the first time during the fifth session. This is an instance of giving new information in the middle of the treatment process. It indicates that therapeutic changes are being made to more serious problems that were central to the discussion of the previous sessions. Thanks to the therapeutic changes in the more severe problems, such secondary grievances find the opportunity to be expressed and dealt with.

life and your career pose limitations to our work, and we are forced to make timetables for you within the same framework.

You need to add another exercise for the new problem you talked about today, along with the three exercises you already do at 7:30, 14:30 and 22. Suppose you have a series of daily routines to do which you know about the previous night. Make a list out of them in your mind. From the beginning of the day, review them in your mind for 5 min every two hours, just like the way they occupy your mind themselves. In these exercises which you do every two hours, you voluntarily recreate and review those thoughts. The reviewed thoughts must be as unpleasant and unwanted as the original ones. Also, you have nothing to do with other times, or with whether the thoughts come or not. This exercise helps you control the annoying, unwanted thoughts.

(It turned out, during the rest of the session, that the client has been trying to fight the thoughts and the anxiety through her own inefficient methods at other times of the day. She was told that her attempts will have no influence, just as they have failed to help her so far. Furthermore, they can interfere with her present treatment and hinder her improvement, slowing down changes. The therapist emphasizes, again, that she must avoid doing such things. She was asked not to do anything other than the exercises.)

C: Both during and after the exercises?

T: Yes, don't do anything to fight the annoying thoughts and the anxiety on your own. Divest yourself of any power in this regard. I wish you had done so from the beginning when I asked you to. If you did, you would have been a lot better right now.[7] The methods you've been using are impractical, as you have experience so far. The only reason you still resort to them is your feeling of urgency and helplessness on the one hand, and the vain hope that they may work this time, and the fear that they may get worse if you don't do what have been doing so far. What you is like a person suffering from a disease, thinking that if he drinks a certain amount of water every day, he will not get cancer, or his cancer will not get worse. You are a physician yourself, so you know quite well that what he does will not have any effects. Doing these things can neither prevent the disease from happening, nor check its progress. This is what you are doing in your own case. You have reached the summit of your problem. You could not be any worse. You have given it enough time to get as worse as possible. The condition does not wait for your permission. It functions independently. If you don't do anything at all, I don't think your problem gets any worse. So, please forget about your own methods so that real treatment can start. What you do is like pulling at the emergency brake while pushing on the gas pedal at the same time. Your personal solution is the emergency brake that prevents the gas pedal from moving the car forward.

C: I did try to recreate everything during the exercises, but at other times I didn't follow your orders. I tried to prevent the thoughts from happening. Now, I know my task is to not do any such thing at other times.

T: Yes, and it's very important.

Session Six

T: It is a pleasure to meet you again. We detected a mistake in your exercises and we discussed how it can be corrected. You were supposed not to make any attempts during the day (any time other than the exercises) to control or avoid annoying thoughts and the anxiety. Please tell me what you did.

C: I did my best to do the exercises. I feel much better now. I felt the stress several times. I felt that my mind was preoccupied with them for only a short time, but I didn't experience extreme tension. I felt much better for the last two weeks, especially the last days of the second week.

T: Hasn't the mistake happen again?

C: No, the interesting point is that when I gave up on fighting them during the day, they didn't happen so often anymore. Both the frequency and the duration of negative thoughts

[7] Behavioral analyses and detailed reports on the performance of the client receiving PTC helps the therapist, as well as the client, to detect any possible mistakes. The mistake made by the client in doing the exercises has slowed down the process of therapeutic change.

have decreased. The worrying and negative thoughts have become much less.

T: Well, it's a good experience from several aspects. First, the actual improvement made is promising, though you must continue doing the exercises. Another point is that sometimes, the wrong method can contribute to the problem further. In this case, it is the mistake we detected the previous session. You were worried that if you don't do what you normally have done, your problem might get worse, which as we saw, it didn't. You actually got better. You and the symptoms of your anxiety are like two people arguing with one another. You believe that if you keep silent and don't argue back, the interlocutor may become more insolent. That is why you keep arguing. What you didn't know was you this is exactly what your opponent wanted, because it gave him an excuse to continue arguing and fighting. But suppose one of the two people arguing is too wise to engage in an argument with a rude, irrational person. The more you begin to neglect the other person, the sooner he will give up.

You need to keep on doing the exercises up to the next session: three times for the first two problems, and every other two hours for the third one. Decrease the exercises by 50% in the second week. Decrease the three times to twice a day, and do the third exercise every four hours. From the third week, do the first exercise only once a day, and keep doing the second exercise every four hours. Keep on doing this last timetable for several weeks up to our next session together. During the interval between our two sessions, there will be social situations in which you must function. You can later report me on how you have done in such situations.

C: Of course, important social situations still scare me and I try to avoid them. Even when I keep my distance from such situations and, for example, do not participate in a conference, my mind is preoccupied with it. It has gotten much better, but it is still there.

T: Well, when you do these focused exercises about your anxiety, and some time passes, one of two things might happen. The first possibility is that the situation loses its negative significance if the base has become weaker or has gone away. This is because the anxiety and stress feed on such bases. The second possibility is that the situation is still scary and annoying to you, for which we will have to make further arrangements.

At this point, the client's husband calls her to ask about the room where the client is having her appointment. It was decided that he will join us. The client added that she had told her husband about her appointment this morning, and had informed him of her problem. The husband had become very upset to learn about a problem he did not know much about before. "We do not hide anything from one another. He has a general idea of my problem. Yet I have never told him the details," the client added.

(The husband enters, the therapist gives him information about the treatment process, how each session unfolds, and the influence this problem can have on other family members and affect the whole family. The help the husband could give to solve his wife's problem was also discussed.)

Before you come, I prescribed for your wife the rest of her timetable. She has to stick to it for two more months. If you have anything to say that can help us adapt and improve the timetable and the exercises, please share it with us. Otherwise, we wait for two months in order to see what our outcomes will be.

Husband: I spent this period of time abroad in order to fulfill my wife's request, actually. She really wanted me to complete my studies. Otherwise, I neither wish personally nor need professionally to receive the education. I said this to make it clear that my first priority in life is her happiness, and I'm ready to do whatever it takes for her to be happy. I am willing to cut my working hours so as to be able to spend more time with my family. Also, I can help her with her career—not in terms of the medical practice, which I know nothing about, but with respect to the management of her daily routines—so that she faces less pressure.

T: Thank you for your cooperation. So, keep on doing the exercises as before up until the next session. We will get help from your husband in the future.

Session Seven

T: It's nice to meet you again. A long time has passed since we had our last session together. Please tell me what you did during this time.

C: I'm better in general and I feel calmer compared to before. Annoying thoughts have decreased, and I feel less stress. There were some real situations as well, which I dealt with having less stress.

T: Have the daily issues that preoccupied your mind decreased?

C: Yes, my mind is freer and everyone around me has noticed the difference. Those who saw me after a while kept telling me "you look so different, you look so happy and calm!".

T: So you have received positive feedback.

C: Yes. Of course they just pay attention to how I look, but I'm feeling it from within. I feel more relaxed, and I have thank you for that.

T: How did you do the exercises?

C: I did them once a day. However, since I couldn't have the optimum focus during the first 10 min, I tried at least twice a day. This way, I had the chance to make up for the mistake I had made the first time.

T: How about conferences and giving speech in front of a crowd?

C: It happened once or twice. It was not like I was able to do it perfectly, but my stress and anxiety was much less than before.

T: Well, that is in line with our prediction. When the source of anxiety is removed, it influences every aspect of your life. What you need to pay attention to right now is that your problem has a long history and deep roots. Therefore, you need to keep on doing the exercises. Fortunately, you are aware of the importance of doing the exercises and you have been able to manage the exercises and do your best. Now, you have a formula which you can use according to the model I prescribed for you here. You also know what the impractical methods are, that you should avoid doing. You must keep doing it for some time, so that the changes and the improvements are stabilized and fixed. This decreases the possibility of relapse. Pay attention that one point was common to all our exercises: welcoming the problems rather than trying to avoid them. If you refer to previous experience, you realize that the more you were afraid of them and tried to avoid them, the stronger an harsher they got and attacked you ever more intensely. You were always the victim in such circumstances. Since you change your method and decided to go to them rather escaping them, they became weaker and weaker and finally they escaped. It was like you were attacking an enemy who had become weak. You should chase them so long that you feel they no longer exist, or are so far that they can't harm you in any way. You are only on the lookout for them. Some enemies cannot be destroyed altogether. We can, however, install and increase reinforcements and be ready so as to deal with any danger coming our way from the enemy.

If anything comes up that makes you feel you need another session, we can arrange one in the future.

The rest of the treatment was carried out within the framework of the PTC model, for dealing with personality problems. Also, a PTC family therapy predicted with respect to the client.

10.3 Assessment of Treatment Outcome and Follow-Up

The course of the treatment was completed in 7 sessions. Assessment of the treatment outcome, which was based on the patients' comments in a graded scale of 0–100 and an open-ended question, indicated 65% recovery. A 20-month follow-up evaluation showed no relapse.

11 Client #9 (Male, 38 Years Old, Married)

11.1 Case Introduction

Mr. MY, a 38-year-old married man, came to the University of Tehran Clinic complaining about panic attacks, fear of death, fear of height, fear of darkness, fear of deep water, and checking gas valve and door locks. The clinical interview based on DSM-5 (APA 2013), confirmed his panic disorder, specific phobias, and compulsive checking. Having a family history of both physical and psychological abuse since his early childhood, MY started experiencing his severe panic attacks, pathological fears and compulsions 16 years ago. MY has already visited psychiatrists and has been taking medication since two years ago. He is living with his wife and his daughter. This is his first visit to receive professional help from a psychotherapist. MY was seen for 6 sessions over a period of 10 weeks.

11.2 Course of Treatment

Session One

Therapist (T): (After greetings and the social stage of the interview) please tell me why you are here.

Client (C): I grew up in a family that taught me fear; fear of ghosts, fear of darkness, fear of heights, fear of fighting and so on were always with me. I wetted my bed up to my teenage years and I was beaten up badly by my parents on account of it. I was not allowed to play outside and with other kids, and if I did, my brothers, who were older than me, would beat me up. I was really cowardly. When I was doing my military service, I suffered from palpitations, but I did not pay much attention to it. At first, it happened every six months. Then, the interval between them decreased and decreased. When an attack of palpitations happens to me, my temples start sweating, my rib cage feels heavy, my hands start trembling, and I panic when I think that I'm having a heart attack. I feel I am losing consciousness and I think that I can only stay alive and get calm by going to a doctor or a hospital immediately.

I manage to keep my spirits high at work. I do artistic work. I do calligraphy and graphic design. I make picture frames and I'm the head color supervisor in a refinery. I have good friends over there, and I spend most of my life there. I work 21 days a month and I'm free for the other 9 days, which I spend with my wife and child.

T: You said that the panic attacks and their corresponding symptoms started during military service. Can you tell me when the attacks happen?

C: I can't tell. They even happen at times when I'm actually happy and laughing. The attack occur suddenly, and when it does, it's almost as if I'm looking death in the eye. After each attack, I feel exhausted for 24 h.

T: Tell me about your other problems.

M. A. Besharat, *Paradoxical Psychotherapy: A Practitioner's Guide*,
University of Tehran Science and Humanities Series,
https://doi.org/10.1007/978-3-031-27717-7_11

C: I'm afraid of the dark. When I'm alone at nights, I leave the lights on. I'm scared of stagnant, deep waters. I'm afraid of heights. At first, when I was working at heights in the refinery, I passed out. Now, I can work at heights up to 40 m, but the panic attacks occurs at that height too.

T: Has there been times when the panic attacks don't happen at heights? Are you still afraid of heights if there are no panic attacks?

C: Yes. Even if there is no panic attack, I'm still afraid of the height.

T: What are the symptoms?

C: My heart starts beating rapidly; I sweat a lot and I can't breathe.

T: You said that it started in your military service, right?

C: I had problems since childhood, but they became what they are now since the military service. It's been 16 years now that I've been dealing with panic attacks and fear of heights, water and darkness. I have recently developed compulsions. When I lock the door, I have to check it several times to make sure. I know it's locked, but I have to check anyway. I did the same with water faucets and gas valves.

T: Do you still do the checking?

C: It has decreased a lot, but I still do it.

T: Have you done anything to cure your problems?

C: I saw a psychiatrist and I took medication for 9 months. But I stopped the medication since it caused me sexual problems (erectile dysfunction). Three months later, the attacks started as severely as ever. It's now been 4 months since I started taking drugs again.

T: Taking into account your working days, you cannot see me to follow my schedule every other two weeks. You have also started taking drugs, again. So, I recommend you to make plans so that we can meet every two weeks, for at least a few sessions. If you manage to do so, you have to stop your medication three months before your next session with me. You can do so after consulting your psychiatrist, or based on your own experience. Then, we can start your treatment.

Session Two

T: It's nice to see you again. A long time has passed since our preliminary session. In that session, we decided that you must make changes to your working schedule so that you can attend a few consecutive sessions with me. It was also decided that you must stop medication three months before the present session. Please, tell me what you did.

C: I stopped the medication right after the previous session. It's been a month since the attacks started more severely than ever. I experienced 12 attacks yesterday, one of them lasting more than 1 h. The symptoms are the same as I told you about, last session. There is this thing, though, that afflicts me very much. When the attack happens, I feel I am dying; and when it ends, I keep worrying about the next attack. I can't have a moment of peace.

T: I asked you to cease the medication 3 months before the session. You ceased them earlier. It's all right, but if you had followed my instruction, the attacks would not have started before our session together. Anyway, we will start our work today. You said that the panic attacks and the fear of death are with you. What about the compulsions?

C: Yes, the compulsion with constant checking is still there.

T: I will give you a task for your panic attacks, which you must do until the next session. First of all, you need to be in a place alone and without anything to interrupt you for 10 min, so that you can focus on the task. Within the 10 min, you must try to feel the attacks, the sweating, the rapid heartbeat and the difficulty in breathing. Your rib cage is heavy and you are about to die in a couple of seconds. What I just described is precisely what you have gone through so many times, unintentionally and unconsciously. This time, I want you to try to experience them intentionally. It's like a bitter drug or a difficult and painful surgery: it is necessary for your treatment and you must tolerate it. What you have to do during the task is to try, honestly and without taking it easy on yourself, to experience all the pain and suffering, as if you are suffering from a real attack. If you manage to do so, you will be treated after 17 years of having to deal with this condition. You may fail to recreate the painful experience of the attacks by 100%, despite your honest attempts; you may only succeed by 50% or less. It is all right, because you have done your best. Despite your diligent efforts, you may not be able to experience any pain whatsoever. You cannot bring yourself to feel the attacks and the fear of impending death. This scenario is also okay, since you have tried your best. There is also one final possibility. You fail to do the task on time. You have forgotten it; you have fallen asleep; you are not alone. If this happens, you simply lose one session for doing the task. You must not try to make up for it, but must wait for the next turn. You either do the tasks precisely on time, or you do not do them at all. Now, we will agree on two 10-min times during the day when you can do the task every day. Remember that the tasks must be done exactly at the hour we decide upon here.

C: I think that 10:30 and 16:30 are fine.

T: Apart from the two 10-min tasks, you mustn't do anything about your problem at other times. You should not try to think or do anything so as to prevent the attacks from happening. You shouldn't try to stop or delay them in any way. The attacks will either happen or not about which we will talk the session after. These two tasks are like two pills you are supposed to take at certain times. You will either get better or worse. Don't think about the outcomes and just do the tasks. You can't both take the pill and wrap a cloth around your head to prevent the headache. You must just take the two pills, precisely at times we have arranged. That's all!

Session Three

T: It is a pleasure to meet you. Tell me what you did.

C: I did the tasks. Of course I couldn't do some of them, because my boss wanted to see me. But I did the rest. When doing the tasks, I couldn't re-experience the actual attacks no matter what I did. It was really difficult to concentrate on those conditions and recreate them.

T: So, you were able to do the tasks to some extent. Tell me about the panic attacks throughout the past two weeks.

C: The attacks have decrease, and they are also different.

T: In what way? Try to tell me in detail what happened.

C: In the past, when I had an attack, my temples became wet with sweat, I couldn't breathe easily, I felt dizzy and it was like I was losing consciousness. Now, my head feels light and it's like blood can't get to my brain; I still feel dizzy, but I think my pressure goes up and down.

T: You said that the attacks have decreased in quantity and changed in quality. What about their severity?

C: Every time I had an attack in the past, I collapsed to the ground in the street or at work. I asked people to take me to the doctor or hospital. Now, I don't ask for help. I take a deep breath and drink a glass of water so the attack goes away. In some cases, when I couldn't take it any longer, I took an Alprazolam or a Propranolol.

T: So now, you don't collapse, or ask for help or go to the hospital?

C: That's right. I don't do them anymore. I manage to keep myself together, since I know that I'm not going to die.

T: How often do the attacks happen every day?

C: About twice a day.

T: You have done a good job so far. You must take the next step more carefully and attentively. Keep on doing the task three times a day, each time for 10 min. In the meantime, try not to take any drugs. Let's assign times for the tasks now.

C: At 1:30, 16:30 and 22:30.

T: And now the compulsive checking. Your compulsion is focused on the water faucet and the door lock in your office. How many times do you lock your office door, or leave the office for work or something?

C: About ten times.

T: All right. Every time you are about to leave, when you lock the door and take some steps away, come back for three times and check the lock and the water faucet. Do this for the first week, and for the second week reduce it to every other time you need to leave. In other words, come back and check the lock and the faucet for only half of the times you leave. See you next session.

Session Four

T: It's nice to see you. Please tell me what you did.

C: I did the tasks. Of course I lost some of them, but I did them as much as I could and I had no attacks within the two weeks. There was only one time when a fleeting feeling came over me. I felt like my head was getting cold. But it was over so soon and I felt no palpitations or difficult breathing or anything.

T: What about the checking?

C: I did them completely for the first week, which really bored and tired me. I was supposed to decrease it during the second week. And now, I am absolutely sure that I have locked the door the first time and I don't check it again. But I've been feeling palpitations in sleep.

T: Do you wake up when they happen?

C: Sometimes.

T: What do you do?

C: I wake up. I take a deep breath. I may drink some water. And I go back to sleep.

T: You mean they subside?

C: Yes.

T: What about when you're awake?

C: I feel less palpitations when I'm awake; but when I go to sleep, they increase.

T: There is the possibility that the palpitations are related to your anxiety. Taking into account the fact that the attacks have recently decreased, we had better wait some more and see whether they will decrease during sleep or not. I don't think you suffer from heart problems, but you can see a cardiologist about it. The next session will be in four weeks. Till then, keep on doing the tasks twice a day (10:30 and 16:30) for 5 min, for the first two weeks; and for the next two weeks, decrease them to once a day (10:30), again for 5 min. Do the compulsive checking tasks on even days, for about 50% of the times you leave your office.

Session Five

T: It's nice to meet you. Tell me what you did.

C: I did the tasks as much as I could. The compulsions have decreased to 15%. I hardly remember I suffered from compulsion in the first place.

T: What about the panic attacks?

C: I had two attacks during the last two weeks. But I felt no fear at all. On one occasion, I felt like I was having a stroke. I drank some water and I went back to normal. On another occasion, I felt a slight fear, which abated soon. There were no more attacks. My palpitations have decreased since 10 days ago. My heartbeat is normal, but I still have slight palpitations. I'm in a much better mood. At work, everybody tells me I've become so much better.

T: We will enter our summer break after this session, which will last until the autumn. You can follow the instructions of the previous session and do the tasks for two more weeks. Then, stop the tasks altogether until our next session together. The healing process will continue throughout the several months we have till the next session. In case the attacks happen again, wait for a few days first. If they don't go away after 5 days, make a plan similar to the one I made for you and start doing it from day 6 and keep doing it for two weeks. This will make the attacks go away. Pay attention that the tasks must be precisely like the ones I gave you. You must assign two times during the day for doing the tasks and then do them exactly at those times.

Session Six

T: About 5 months have passed since our last session together. Please, tell me what you did.

C: Everything went on perfectly. I no longer have compulsions. And the attacks didn't occur, so I didn't need to make a new timetable.

(During the rest of the session, the patient talked about sexual relations with his wife. It was decided that he and his wife should visit the therapist on another occasion for that.)

11.3 Assessment of Treatment Outcome and Follow-Up

The course of the treatment was completed in 6 sessions. Assessment of the treatment outcome, which was based on the patients' comments in a graded scale of 0–100 and an open-ended question, indicated 90% recovery. A 3-year follow-up evaluation indicated that there was no relapse.

12 Client #10 (Female, 33 Years Old, Single)

12.1 Case Introduction

Miss. RE 33 years old, single, was referred to the University of Tehran Clinic because of her social anxiety, relatively low mood and shaky self-confidence. The symptoms of the disorder have existed on since her childhood and adolescence. However, they have become more severe, annoying and dominant since two years ago and have disrupted her personal and professional life. Her symptoms fulfilled the DSM-5 (APA 2013) criteria for social anxiety disorder including severe stress at social situations among colleagues, fear of being addressed by others and avoidance behaviors. The patient's social anxiety is so much that she has difficulty going to a shop and buying things: "Even while buying a bottle of milk, or when using my credit card to pay for things, I feel so stressed that my hands shake noticeably." Among her family members, her mother suffers from anxiety disorder, too. RE does not take medication at present and this is her first visit for psychological treatment. RE was seen for 3 sessions over a period of 4 weeks.

12.2 Course of Treatment

Session One

Therapist (T): (After greetings and the social stage of the interview) Please tell me why you are here.

Client (C): I have a history of anxiety with social anxiety being more prominent, a relatively low mood and low self-confidence. These problems, both along with and against some of my other abilities and characteristics (my educational accomplishments and my calm appearance), have impressed others, including some of my own patients. Therefore, it was under my control to some extent. Until recently, things happened that made me realize it was no longer under my control and started to worry me. I had a similar experience two years ago. It was the fourth year of my residency training when I fell into a serious depression that affected my performance. It was so bad that I was only able to pass my exams with difficulty at the end of the fourth year, while I had been elected the top resident at the first year, and got the best rank again at the third year. After two months, I got myself together and I was able to pass the national board examination, which is a difficult exam (the patient, who was clearly anxious from the beginning of the session, starts crying at this point). I'm sorry!

T: It's okay!

C: Time went by, and this low mood and anxiety was with me. At the end of my training, I was given a good position where I was really successful. Although everyone predicted that I would stay in that position for at least two more years, I suddenly announced that I can no longer work there. I couldn't continue anymore despite my good situation and the constant demands of my bosses. When I came back, I had two months

M. A. Besharat, *Paradoxical Psychotherapy: A Practitioner's Guide*, University of Tehran Science and Humanities Series, https://doi.org/10.1007/978-3-031-27717-7_12

to reinvigorate myself because I was free. But life was too difficult. I didn't let anybody know about my problems, but it was really difficult to bear (starts crying uncontrollably). I never thought I'd end up like this. I always thought I'd gotten all better.

T: Sometimes, the mere recounting of some bitter experience, which might have been resolved, can be really upsetting. Well, what happened within the two months?

C: Yeah! The social anxiety increased in the two months. It was even difficult for me to go shopping. It was torture! I wasn't like this all the time, though. But when it happened, it was really upsetting. Or, one of my professors who has always been good to me, invited to take part in some surgeries. I felt no stress to be in the surgery room, or to stand beside my professor. But the minute I left the surgery room to take off my costume and socialize with my colleagues, I got so stressed. If they asked me a question, or if I wanted to ask something, I became seriously stressed. I felt that I must do something about my problem.

T: So you feel social anxiety at work, while socializing with colleagues and when shopping. What was it like during shopping?

C: It's really weird during shopping. I think it might be because I am upset. Even when I want to pay for a bottle of milk, or get my credit card, my hands shake visibly. And it's really strange to me.

T: What are the consequences of the anxiety? Apart from the handshaking?

C: Handshaking, and palpitations in face to face conversations! And sometimes, when I'm talking on the phone, I feel I'm short of breath.

T: How long have you had such anxiety?

C: Such severe anxiety is new and totally unprecedented. But I've had mild anxiety since childhood.

T: So you've had some background in anxiety. You have accumulated experience over the years. You have greater abilities, mental power and reasoning. Therefore, you must have the anxiety under greater control, but it's gotten worse, right?

C: I can't explain it. My job is a really stressful one. Compared to my job, my life isn't stressful at all. I can't understand why this must happen.

T: You mentioned something about depression. Can you tell me more?

C: Low mood, lack of motivation, unhappiness which has usually been mild but became severe in my last year as a resident and disrupted my work; we were getting ready for the board examination and I hadn't been able to use any of the rotations offered to me, which was really bad.

T: Have those low moods been with you all the time?

C: Doctor, there are traces of it in my personality, but it has never had a continuous, chronic state. Maybe, I have never been a relaxed and easygoing person. But I wasn't a solitary, clinically depressed person with lots of problems in my life and work, either. Let's say my clinical presentation did not match with different types of anxiety. However, within the two months, I must have been able to do something, but I felt myself incapable of going to the university and starting a series of time-consuming paper-work.

T: Do you think this lack of ability to take care of certain things has been due to depression or anxiety, or both?

C: Both.

T: Now that you are here, with some anxieties having been intensified, do you think you have depression too?

C: I thought there wasn't, but there is. I'm not dealing with occupational stress, and I have a good family. But I don't have a mood stability.

T: Now, you are studying to get ready for a specialty. It means that you are working harder than medium, is that right?

C: That is right.

T: Do you live with your family?

C: Yes.

T: Is there anyone like you in your family?

C: My mother suffers from anxiety too, but she is not like me. I'm an introvert and I try not to show or express my feelings. My other family members are not like this. They're easygoing.

T: You mean you are introvert everywhere, even in your own home and among other family members?

C: Yes.

T: Well, is there anything else?

C: No.

T: Let's deal with them one at a time, right? (both laughing).

I make a timetable for your anxiety, the most recent type of anxiety you've had; and then we move on from there. You must do the exercises I give you precisely according to this timetable. In each exercise unit, you situate yourself for up to 10 min at a proper place, where you can have concentration to do the exercise, and imagine all the conditions that have recently given you anxiety and try to recreate and re-experience them. The more these recreations resemble the actual experience of anxiety, the more complete your treatment will be. In fact, in this exercise you must play a role that matches reality completely, both formally and in terms of content. In other words, the anxious state and the corresponding symptoms such as palpitations, hand tremor, shaky voice and short breath must be precisely similar to the real ones. Also, you must forget about all the arguments and assumptions we made here while doing the exercises, because they can get in the way of doing the exercises the right way. For instance, it is okay for you, here, to consider your anxiety while shopping as something ridiculous. But when you are doing the exercises, you must refrain from making similar comments and just focus on doing the exercise. That's not the time to reason and argue. You just have to let negative emotions overwhelm you. It's even useful to dig in the past and try to find things that can create anxiety and stress in you. You need to do this exercise at certain times during the day. Our next session will be in two weeks. For the first week, you must do the exercise three times a day, each time for 10 min maximum. For the second week, you will do it twice a day. You must start tomorrow. Now, give me three times during the day when you can do the tasks.

C: For the first week, 10:30, 17:00 and 20:00; and for the second week, 10:30 and 17:00.

T: In doing the exercises, you have done a complete job when you can recreate the anxiety and depression as I said. You may not be able to recreate them by 100%, though, and only manage by 50%, or fail altogether. No matter what happens, it's all right as long as you make an honest effort. You may also fail to do the exercise on time, for any possible reasons. If this happens, you mustn't try to make up for the lost exercise by doing it at some other time. Therefore, you either do the exercises on time, or you don't do them at all. For the first three to four days, you had better not put yourself in real-life stress and anxiety-inducing situations. But after that, you must welcome them. For instance, if you have so far avoided going shopping due to your problem and have asked others to do it for you, after four days you must do it yourself. Also, when you put yourself in real situations, don't try to give yourself hope and lift your spirits by telling yourself you will manage this time. No! Quite the reverse, you must enter the situation with the expectation that you will experience great anxiety again.

Session Two

T: Nice to meet you again. Tell me what you did, please.

C: I'm much better, compared to before. I did most of the exercises for the first week. I had to go on a trip during the second week, so I couldn't do some of the exercises. I was able to recreate the anxiety by 60%. During the first week, although I focused on anxiety, I became more sad than anxious.

T: Did that happen while doing the exercises?

C: Mainly after them, immediately after each exercise. It was a short spell, and went away quickly. When I gave my problem some more thought, I believe that what I told you about is not the problem per se, but it's my inability to manage my emotions and affects that is the problem. Take shopping and conversations, for instance. If it's just shopping or conversing, there's no problem. But, if the communication becomes a little deeper (if it becomes emotional), it embarrasses me and creates anxiety. Then, I feel depressed due to my problem, and the depression worsens everything all over.

T: So, if any of your relationships takes an emotional or romantic turn, it creates anxiety in you. Is that right?

C: Yes, and the deeper the emotion is, the greater the anxiety will be.

T: Well, let's look at the problem from this point of view. Have you ever been involved in a romantic relationship in your life?

C: Not seriously.

T: I want to know what happens then.

C: Can you explain?

T: Have you ever felt love for anybody? Have you ever developed an either deep or shallow friendly or romantic relationship with anyone? If yes, I would like to know how you have behaved in such a case.

C: As long as I can remember, since high school and the teenage years, I always suppressed such feelings within me. I'm not like that anymore. But, if a case comes up, it creates anxiety and stress in me.

T: You don't feel comfortable with such relationships and friendships?

C: Maybe I act like it's okay and I can manage it somehow. But I get really anxious and embarrassed, inside.

T: Anxiety and embarrassment aside, anyone grows up in a specific environment with different beliefs and values around her. Someone is brought up as shy, someone with a feeling of guilt and someone else with negative emotions. Anyone looks at life differently, but they all end up marrying someone. What do you think about marriage?

C: I am okay with this process and the marriage. I have a problem with having to choose. I don't feel an urgent need to get married right now, because I see the huge responsibility of married life, and the limitations it imposes on one's life. And my emotional needs are satisfied within my family of origin. It's of different type, but it is. Under such circumstances, it's really difficult for me to be able to choose someone.

T: Therefore, the need is there, and your attitude is positive. However, the criteria, responsibilities and related difficulties have created an obstacle. So, in your opinion, the main problem is the emotional aspect of your relationships. Now, tell me more about the emotional atmosphere in your family.

C: It's very good.

T: How many people are there in your family?

C: I have two brothers plus my mom and dad. Everything's fine, and we live in a pleasant atmosphere. Despite this, I prefer not to talk about such matters with my family, because it will upset them. Recently, when we were all together, I suddenly burst out crying. It had never happened before, and I'd never had such a reaction in similar situations. And it made my family really upset.

T: When did this happen?

C: During the first week after our previous session together, and they were very worried about me. They tried to soothe me and wanted to know what had happened.

T: And you said that this had never happened before?

C: No, that was the first time. It's funny, since before it happened, I'd said in a job interview that I'd never cried in front of a group of people and never would.

T: And when you were with your family at home, you started crying?

C: It was horrible. I couldn't help myself. It was like a sudden attack. Everyone was talking normally, and my mood changed suddenly.

T: Were you talking about anything special?

C: No, it was nothing special. They were surprised and kept wondering what had caused it. Were you reminded of something, they asked. And they were really upset that I couldn't talk with them and unburden myself to them. It made them upset, as well.

T: Well, let me recapitulate your scenario so far: there is some history of anxiety which is, as you put it, relation to emotional issues. And you confirmed that you've always had a low mood. We human beings have different aspects, abilities and weaknesses. Sometimes, one aspect develops greatly. For instance, we get really good in education, and turn into a really successful and outstanding person. On the other hand, other aspects of our personality don't get the chance to grow, such as emotional growth. When it comes to family and the society, we have other people's expectations that can be really important to us. For instance, people imagine that a successful and educated person must necessarily lead a successful emotional and romantic life. Well, someone who is fully developed in one aspect, but has remained underdeveloped in another, faces serious limitations. She encounters a great void, followed by feelings of incompetence and inadequacy which can question the person's self-worth and self-confidence. It's almost as if she has been oblivious of something for years. She has improved rapidly and successfully in one aspect, but has remained practically underdeveloped in another aspect. She wakes up, and realizes that she really needs that other aspect, which is lacking. The psyche is suddenly helpless, although temporarily. This is your situation now, which needs to be reorganized. Now, the more the person facing the void is aware of her problem, the greater her pain will be; this is the case for you.

C: That's right.

T: And there is another problem. You cannot solve this equation with reasoning and rational arguments. This problem is a completely emotional and affective one, which is exactly what makes it a clinical condition difficult to either understand or solve. The person suffering from this condition thinks to herself and sees that there is nothing in her past, or her education that calls for such a situation. She is totally puzzled.

Taking into account what we talked about today, we need to adapt the exercises a little bit. Keep on doing exercises three times a day, each time for 10 min. Imagine emotional affairs: start from the surface and gradually go deeper. Bring to life the emotions and anxieties that you normally feel and re-experience them. You need to do this exercise for a while. I also would like to know what happens in your family, when you do these exercises. A question has been left unanswered in your family. Everyone, plus yourself, would like to know why you were so upset that day. We need to interpret it in some way.

I would also like to know more about your personal, romantic world. Such a world is filled with emotions and affects that are problematic to you. Such emotions and affects are both sexual and asexual. In one form, it is an interactional, two-person world, and in another form, it is personal and intrinsic. Does such a world exist within you?

C: I guess I have the potential for it, but it's not active.

T: That's one of the things that needs to be activated. The question is, why hasn't it become active before? It's one of the natural needs of human beings. It begins in people from a certain age and we can see its signs from the outside. Now, if it hasn't emerged in someone, we must ask why? In answering this question, we will probably arrive at the psychological roots of the problem. Is there some inhibition at work in the person's mind in this respect? Are there conflicts at work? And similar questions. When you say that you have the potential, but it's not active, it means that something is wrong. However, there is also a paradox to what you say. If there is the potential, it must show itself under any circumstances and be activated on its own, just like it is in many people. Why doesn't it work in your case? Can we say that there is no potential? I don't think this is the answer, since why would the person think of it in the first place? Can we say that certain situations have served as obstacles to it? If yes, we must try to identify those situations and deal with them.

In other words, what we see in others as the desire to have emotional affairs, which is the outer indication of such a potential, must have some sort of inner indication. There must be something inside the individual, something active that is first experienced personally and then manifests itself in terms of an interpersonal relationship. If there is no such dynamic inner world, we must ask why? What has inhibited and suppressed its emergence? If it emerges from within, it can serve as a strong and natural antidepressant. If it doesn't emerge, we must ask why?

C: Well, it hasn't emerged. The problem has nothing to do with my family. But, when I look back on my past, to the time when such feelings and desires were activated in others my age, I remember that I always suppressed them, somehow.

T: And since they have been suppressed for a long time, it's folder has been closed and has remained closed. It is difficult and problematic for it to be opened again. The reason I discussed these issues is that we need, first, to work on these feelings and affects from within and activate them, so that we can then bring them in relations with other people without causing any further problems. Now, in order to activate this inner world, you must get help from anything you know can be effective. Work on it until the next session when we can talk about it and see whether it's necessary to give you a special timetable or not.[1]

Session Three

T: Hello. Pleasure to meet you. Tell me what you did.

C: Last session, we mainly talked about controlling and managing feelings and affects. My exercise included recreating similar cases that give me stressful emotions. It was an interesting experience. I had this job to do, which I was postponing due to my problem. After three days of doing the exercise, I got ready for a job interview, which was also emotionally significant for me. It was perfect, since I felt no stress before or during the interview. And, after the interview I felt great. I was happy about this good experience for a couple of days, and I didn't feel the need to do the exercise. My happiness decreased afterwards, but my stress has decreased in general. That's how it went (in this session, unlike the first session, the patient spoke in a happy, calm tone).

As for the exercise related to romantic issues, I was only willing to do it only once within the past two weeks. And that was during the time I was happy after the interview. Although I was supposed to do it, I didn't feel like doing it.

T: How was it that one time? Did you feel anything?

C: Well, I searched the net for a romantic scene, and I found one. That's all. I didn't do anything else.

T: It's good enough for a start. The more you have similar experience the better. It can help to resolve your present conflicts and make you active in this respect. This kind of experience helps you understand the problem better. You mentioned something last session about which we did not talk. You said that you have experienced some sort of inhibition and sexual suppression since your teenage years. Is that right?

C: Yes, by myself. I don't deny it.

T: That's right. As an educated adult, you reason that there is such a need which is important. You say it and you agree with anyone else who says so. You will also add that it is necessary for developing a couple relationship and having a family. It's all easy to say. But, when it comes to actually doing something, it is necessary that the motivation comes from inside. The problem is that it doesn't. There are two assumptions: first, the individual can be sexually active if it is not for the inhibitions that have been with her since childhood. According to the second assumption, the individual might be sexually frigid. We must see which assumption is more probable.

C: I think they're both true, although I guess the first assumption is more probable.

T: Well, you have to start being sexually active. You have done a preliminary job for a start, But you need to be more active in this regard. The engine that hasn't worked in years, cannot be turned on easily. It needs to be taken care of. Sexual desire can be activated through various stimuli. You have your personal taste, preference and desire and there are specific stimuli that can turn you on. Since you are single, you must deal with it alone. You said that there is the desire and the capability to engage in such personal sexual experiment and there are no personal inhibitions against it. Therefore, you need to have romantic and sexual experience

[1] Analytic doctrines are used a lot in the PTC model. The level and depth of such doctrines differs according to each individual patient's level of understanding and reasoning. The therapeutic goal of these doctrines is first to prepare the ground for encouraging the patient to carry out the exercises correctly; especially those exercises which, due to cultural and educational reasons, might need something more than mere prescription. Such doctrines, especially in cases when the goal is to change personality traits of the patient, are particularly important and prominent.

(seeing, touching, being turned on, reaching orgasm and so on) so that the sex engine can start. The plans we have made for you have had messages for us. For example, that interview told you who you are, what you can do and what consequences you must expect of similar situations. In general, you can get to know yourself and your problems better. According to such an understanding, you can take the next steps with greater preparation. Part of the exercises you have to do next includes trying to turn on your sex engine. In terms of family relations, you said things about your mom and dad which were pretty positive. I would like to know more, however.

C: My father is an introvert, although I'm still more introvert than he is. My mother, however, is an extrovert and sociable.

T: How is their relationship?

C: It's fine, and they are sort of accustomed to one another (no more mentionable information was made about parents and their relationship).

T: Well, you have shown great motivation for educational success. You are now getting ready for your specialty. So far, you have spent all your time and energy in this respect. Also, your introversion has also made you distance yourself from others. Your emotions and affects, which have so far been stagnant, need to be activated. We agreed that you need to turn on your emotions and affects, and your sex engine. You said that you feel, at times, that you don't need any more exercises. You are doing these exercises to re-experience stress and anxiety. However, the fact that you don't experience them any more while doing the exercises doesn't mean that you should stop doing them. Therefore, you definitely need to keep on doing the anxiety exercises. Continue doing it once a day, for 5 min. When can you do it?

C: 10:30 would be fine.

T: As for romantic and sexual exercises, it is necessary that you find stronger stimuli. Also, you need to do this exercise at least once a week. As you move on, such emotions must become more active. When they do, you need to increase the exercises and do them at least twice a week.

C: Do you recommend anything in particular?

T: This is mainly a personal issue. What can be both sexually arousing and acceptable for each individual? For a man, a picture of a woman can serve this purpose, or a film. For a woman, it might be different. Now, each individual does certain things along with using such aids. Since you are doing this alone, options range from sexual fantasies to sexual stimulation. As I said, this is mainly a personal issue which you need to experience on your own.

The rest of the treatment was defined within the PTC framework for personality disorders, plus sex-therapy.

12.3 Assessment of Treatment Outcome and Follow-Up

The course of the treatment was completed in 3 sessions. Assessment of the treatment outcome, which was based on the patients' comments in a graded scale of 0–100 and an open-ended question, indicated 100% recovery. A 30-month follow-up evaluation showed no relapse.

13 Client #11 (Male, 26 Years Old, Single)

13.1 Case Introduction

NK, a 26-year-old single man, was referred to the University of Tehran Clinic by a counseling center. NK explained his symptoms thus in the first session: “Following an unprotected sexual intercourse, I was afraid I might have contracted AIDS. I have had tests twice so far, which said that I am HIV negative. As time goes on, however, I feel more and more anxious and scared and I constantly check my body for AIDS symptoms. Whenever I hear anything about this illness, I feel really, really bad. My sleep is disturbed, I have lost my concentration, I have become short-tempered and irritable, I feel indifferent about everything and I have lost all motivation”. The clinical interview based on DSM-5 (APA 2013), confirmed the existence of illness anxiety disorder. He was also diagnosed to have symptoms of depressive disorder. The disorders have had a great impact on his job, interpersonal relationships; and it is a great burden on quality of life. NK had no history of taking medication and does not use drugs now. This is his first visit to receive psychological treatment. NK was seen for 5 sessions over a period of 8 weeks.

13.2 Course of Treatment

Session One

Therapist (T): (After greetings and the social stage of the interview) tell me a little bit about what brings you here today.

Client (C): My problem is obsessive thinking. I have already visited two doctors but it was useless. My second psychologist referred me to you.

T: What do you mean by obsession?

C: I had an unprotected sexual relationship recently. After two or three months, I became worried about having AIDS. I got an HIV test but the result was negative. Seven months later, I went somewhere else but the result was still negative and they told me not to worry about it but I think I have HIV symptoms. About three months ago, when I got my second HIV test, my fears and worries increased. My sleep has been disturbed, I can't concentrate anymore and I've become restless and aggressive. Lately, I went to a Counselling Center for two or three sessions; they were not able to help me so they referred me to you. I guess I've a history of obsession. I remember when I was in high school, I used to doodle on the arm of the chair or paint it. I still

M. A. Besharat, *Paradoxical Psychotherapy: A Practitioner's Guide*,
University of Tehran Science and Humanities Series,
https://doi.org/10.1007/978-3-031-27717-7_13

have this habit. Suddenly I realize I've drawn things here and there! I don't know whether they are related to each other or not.

T: When did you start worrying about AIDS?

C: Since last year. Exactly last summer.

T: After you had these worries, you went to get an HIV test twice and your problem got worse and worse. Is that right?

C: Yes. Especially after the second HIV test, it became worse.

T: And now you are worried about being HIV positive, right?

C: Yes.

T: Tell me about its symptoms?

C: My sleep is disturbed; I constantly check the symptoms on me and as soon as I read something about this illness, I feel terrible.

T: You mentioned your past and talked about high school and the doodling. Was there anything else before you worried about having AIDS?

C: No. There wasn't anything but now this issue has obsessed my mind. Another thing is that I've become so aggressive.

T: How is your aggression expressed?

C: I lose my temper too quickly, at home. I've become indifferent to everything. I feel bad about this indifference; I've lost all my motivation.

T: When did your indifference and lack of motivation begin?

C: I used to be like this in the past but it was temporary. After this happened to me last December (four months ago), my problem continued and got worse.

T: You don't sleep well anymore, you wake up in the morning badly, and you are indifferent and unmotivated, right? And all this began since last December?

C: Yes. I've had these feelings before but they were periodic.

T: What do you mean by periodic?

C: It depended on the conditions. For example, I did terrible on the MA exam and I got depressed and I didn't feel well then; at the end of my graduate years, there was a time when I felt very bad.

T: What happened then?

C: I fell in love with a girl who didn't love me back.

T: So, all these happened in the past, and then they automatically disappeared?

C: Yes. They gradually disappeared when I participated in social activities, and got together with friends. But this last one has not gone away yet.

T: Are you stuck in it?

C: Yes I am. I'm stuck in it very badly.

T: In the past, you didn't have any worries about the illness; you had occasionally some depressive states and they gradually disappeared but this time, these depressive states are paired with your worry about having AIDS and for this reason, they have lingered on and have annoyed you. Is that right?

C: Yes. It's been hindering me.

T: Have you gone to a psychiatrist for treating these depressive states?

C: No. I've just gone to two psychologists and the second one recommended you to me.

T: Are there any other problems besides your depressive states and worries about having AIDS?

C: No. there is nothing special. If I happen to remember anything else, I'll tell you about it.

T: No problem. If you happen to remember anything, you can tell me either in this session or in the next sessions because we are going to have a couple of more sessions. You should keep in mind that many young men of your age do what you did last year but they don't become like you. Do they?

C: No they don't.

T: They definitely don't.

C: I'm sure none of them would become like me.

T: That's the point. There are at least 100 people who do what you've done but they don't become so much worried like you. Even if one of them becomes worried, he gets an HIV test and when he finds out there is no problem, he moves on; but you were not able to do so even when two test results proved you wrong. The meaning behind all this is that you are sensitive but it's not related to what you experienced; if it weren't because of your oversensitivity, then out of 100 people, one might feel just like you. Even if it is assumed that the risk is more than 70 percent, all the 100 people will get a test and when their results turn out to be negative, they will live their lives and may even experience sexual activities just like before. But you were not able to do so and your inner sensitivity has entrapped you; this is not related to that experience at all. Keep in mind that if it had been related to that experience, then the problem would have been solved by the test result; the test result could have convinced you, but because your problem was not caused by that experience, the test result turned out to be useless. Now I will make a plan for you to decrease your inner sensitivity.

I'll make a series of tasks for you to do. It takes you 7–10 min to do every task. What you need to do is to stay in a quiet place where no one can disturb you and focus on all the thoughts that have been bothering you lately. You should recreate all those thoughts about having AIDS and its consequences and symptoms. You should experience them with all their bitterness and worries. Try to recreate all those issues you have mentioned in the session and all the things you may have forgotten to say. In other words, try to recreate and re-experience exactly the thoughts that automatically obsessed your mind with the same degree and intensity. There are some possibilities that may occur in doing the tasks. You may succeed in recreating the thoughts exactly like the ones that automatically happened to you. If this happens, this will be the best result. But it is possible that you try your best to feel as real as possible but the result turns out to be different. For example, they might be just 40 or 50% similar to the reality. If this happens, there will be no problem because you have tried your best. There may be times when you try your hardest, but those thoughts and feelings do not enter your mind. Still, there will be no problem because you have made efforts to do so. There is another possibility that might happen to you. You should do these tasks on certain hours that we both agree on. If you happen to sleep or forget the time, or if you are not able to find the right place and, as a result, miss a task due to any reasons, you have to skip the task and try not to make up for it. You can't make up for it because these tasks are either done on the due time or not done at all. This is an instruction for you. The tasks might be bitter but they are simple because you should recreate the thoughts and feelings that have been bothering you day and night for the last year and that you have been very well familiar with. Now let's draw a timetable. Think about three different times during the day when you can do the tasks. These occasions should fit in with your daily life. For the first week you ought to do the tasks three times a day and for the second week, twice a day.

C: It will be 8:00, 16:00, and 23:00 for the first week and 8:00 and 23:00 for the second week.

T: All right. The timetable is now established. You don't have to do anything tonight and from tomorrow morning on, your first task will start. Another thing you have to pay attention to is the point that what we just talked about is all the plan you must stick to. You should not do anything else during the day. It means that you should not try to help yourself in any other ways, such as trying to avoid these thoughts in other situations. You should not do anything else. We will talk about whatever happens during these two weeks.

Session Two

T: Welcome. Please, tell me about what you have done during the last two weeks.

C: I was able to do 80% of the tasks. At the first session, I forgot to tell you that my obsession revolved around the contaminated needle that I thought they used to take my blood for the HIV test. This thought hurt me really bad. So I thought about it very much in the tasks. On top of that, whenever I catch a cold, I think about this illness (AIDS) more often and I become ill. I've already had sinus infection and when it gets worse, my mind becomes obsessed with AIDS and after that I feel terrible.

T: So you have done the tasks in the last two weeks. How have you been in these two weeks?

C: I feel I've become better now. When I recreated the thoughts myself, they wouldn't automatically haunt me anymore. I mean the thoughts obsess my mind less than before. On the other hand, I tried very hard to bring the thoughts to my mind but they didn't (starts smiling). All in all, the number of intrusive thoughts decreased but they did not disappear altogether. They occasionally come to my mind and bother me.

T: How much do you think the number of thoughts have decreased?

C: I guess they have decreased by 30–40%.

T: You have taken the first step very strongly. According to my instruction, you entered one or two forgotten issues into the tasks. To continue the tasks for the next two weeks, you need to do them four times for the first week and three times for the second week. However, the 7–10 min duration of the task will decrease to 5 min at the most. At what time do you like to do the tasks for the next two weeks?

C: At 9:00, 13:00, 17:00, and 23:00 for the first week and at 9:00, 17:00, and 23:00 for the second week. Doctor, I have a question. I'd like to know what will happen to my depression and bad mood.

T: Let's suppose that all or some of your problems are caused by your worries about having this condition. Let's wait and solve this problem first and then we will find out what remains. Nothing important may remain in the next two weeks.

Session Three

T: You are welcome. Tell me what you've done and what happened.

C: I completed less tasks compared to before. I guess I've done about 70% and the result was good.

T: You have done the tasks by 70%. What about the result?

C: I've got better by 40–50%.

T: You mean the presence of these thoughts and worries have decreased by 40–50%.

C: Yes. The idea that the needle was contaminated now sounds meaningless and irrational. Whatever I focus on fades away and disappears. I still have lack of motivation and low concentration. Of course I've always had difficulty concentrating and some of my friends noticed and thought I was being indifferent to them and they got annoyed. I think this problem is not related to this illness because it's been always with me; it's not affected my studies but since my mind was obsessed with this illness (AIDS), I lose my concentration more often.

T: There are two issues here; one is your personality trait which is regarded as a personal difference and cannot be considered a problem. Usually people are fine and accept these traits and even if they really want to change them, they can succeed to some extent. The other issue is about dealing with your worries, which we decided to wait and see what remains after this problem is solved. It's still too soon to deal with another issue. There is no need to do that now.

But for the next session, we need to have sessions not every two weeks but every month. This time interval will show more clearly whether these consequences will disappear or not. For the first two weeks, you should do the tasks three times a day and for the next two weeks, do them twice a day. Let's draw the timetable. At what time will you do them?

C: At 9:00, 19:00, and 23:00 for the first two weeks and at 9:00 and 23:00 for the second two weeks. Doctor, are there any other tasks I should do?

T: No, these tasks will suffice.

C: Yes. I think this is working for me.

Session Four

T: You are welcome. How is everything with you?

C: I feel better. The timetable was drawn for four weeks; and now, I feel better.

T: How much would that be in percentage?

C: I can't say I felt 100% well but I felt better by 85–90%. There are some exceptions but generally the thoughts of needles, and the symptoms have lost their meanings. The few obsessive thoughts, which used to hurt me, do not haunt me anymore. I've been feeling better; I can concentrate more, I have higher motivation; I was able to start working; I generally feel comfortable.

T: Seemingly, these are the last moments of your problem. Comparing it to a game, I suppose it's over and I'll tell you how to handle the game so as to get all the points. Is there anything else I can be of help?

C: One of the problems that have bothered me so much and held me back in life is my low self-confidence. I think I'm strong in so many fields but this low self-confidence has always kept me behind. My main weakness in life is having a low confidence.

T: How does this low confidence show itself?

C: For instance, if I happen to discuss something in a group, it becomes very difficult for me to talk. Although I prepare myself for the topic I'm going to talk about, I can't explain it right. I don't have any problems among friends, but in formal settings, I get nervous.

T: Do you usually feel nervous before talking about things?

C: Yes.

T: And then during the session, it reaches its peak. Is that right?

C: Yes. I usually try to avoid these sessions and escape them. This is something within me that makes me think I can't do anything, a feeling of inferiority. I took my bachelor's degree in X University and got my MA degree in Z University; I feel my friends were able to show other people what they were capable of doing while I wasn't.

T: You told me you had this low self-confidence and inferiority feelings in certain situations. How does it show itself in your relationships with girls?

C: This feeling is more intense when I'm with girls, like when I was in university. Girls and boys would talk together, but not me. Especially during my freshman year, I got shy and didn't know what to say. As time passed, I got better but I still think I have problems.

T: These gradual changes might be because of getting older and having more experience; they were not systematic and purposeful ways to solve your problem. Is that right?

C: Yes.

T: Have you noticed what makes this condition (low confidence, inferiority feelings and difficulty speaking in public) better or worse?

C: No. I don't remember what made it better or worse.

T: Is there anything else besides low self-confidence and inferiority feelings?

C: Generally I am a conservative person. I don't take risks. I'm afraid of experiencing new things like traveling to new places; this trait is common among all my family members.

T: Look! We need several more sessions to solve this problem and we are near the holidays, so now is not a good time to start. We will deal with that problem right after the summer.

We are going to have a long holiday. You need to do the tasks once a day for another week; the week after that, you should do the tasks only on even days; from the third week on, stop doing the tasks. If everything is okay and no problem shows up, you can go on like that till October, when we meet again; however, if something comes up, and you have the problem once again, give yourself five days to check whether it is temporary or not, and if the problem doesn't go away and lingers on for five days, do the tasks on the fifth day based on the instructions I gave you. For example, you can make plans on the fifth day and draw a timetable to do the tasks three times a day, with five minutes for each time. I'm sure you will be able to do so if it becomes necessary. This treatment plan is similar to your pills; you don't need them now but if conditions change, you can take them in the future.

Session Five

T: So it's been four months since our last session. In the last session we saw general improvements regarding your worries about getting the disease and later you talked about your low self-confidence which we put off till now. Let's hear about your report on the problem and let me know how you have been for the last four months.

C: The progress continued and there were no serious problems. However, at times, when my sinus infection gets worse, I become worried because both AIDS and sinus infection have similar symptoms; but my worries and anxieties don't last and disappear quickly. I was curious to make plans for myself and do the tasks once again to see what would happen. I did so and I found it helpful and useful one more time. I consider the problem solved and, in fact, I don't see it as a problem anymore and the thoughts that haunted me day and night now sound trivial and funny. Now I'd like to work on my self-confidence and the ability to speak in public.

T: So, apparently we are done with your first problem and by this personal experience, you've realized that you don't have to worry about the relapse and even if the problem shows up again, you know how to deal with it. For sure, as time goes by, these few intrusive thoughts will disappear too and you won't experience even these temporary problems.

The rest of the treatment revolved around PTC formulation for personality problems.

13.3 Assessment of Treatment Outcome and Follow-Up

The course of the treatment was completed in 5 sessions. Assessment of the treatment outcome, which was based on the patients' comments in a graded scale of 0–100 and an open-ended question, indicated 100% recovery. A 28-month follow-up evaluation revealed no relapse.

14 Client #12 (Female, 24 Years Old, Married)

14.1 Case Introduction

Mrs. SS a 24-year-old married woman referred to the University of Tehran Clinic with her husband mainly complaining of serious worries and anxieties concerning both structural and functional pathologies of her heart and brain. The clinical interview confirmed her symptoms as illness anxiety disorder based on DSM-5 (APA 2013). SS's illness anxiety disorder started about 4 years ago shortly after her marriage. She said "*I constantly had blood and urine tests and so on. Then it was my heart. I had electrocardiography which showed nothing. But I couldn't feel relaxed*". All these have become worse as time goes on. Her husband described part of their communication as: "*All we talk about at home is health and different types of diseases. She keeps asking me to check her pulse and see if it's normal or not*". Taking medications including Fluoxetine and Chlordiazepoxide has not help SS to get rid of the disorder and this is her second visit for a psychological treatment. SS was seen for 7 sessions over a period of 9 weeks.

14.2 Course of Treatment

Session One

Therapist (T): (After greetings and the social stage of the interview) Please, tell me why you are here.

Husband (H): My wife thinks she has some illnesses. For example, she thinks that her heart doesn't beat, or that her head is light, or blood doesn't get to his brain, or she keeps thinking her body is not like everyone else's. She is always afraid these problems end in her death. Or, she says "I can't come to that party, because I may feel bad and I can't have access to an ambulance or a hospital, there."

(When the husband, who has been the sole speaker, finishes, the therapist turns to the wife and asks her to talk about her problems, personally.)

Client (C): I was a really lively and happy girl. A couple of years ago, my cousin passed away due to cancer. I felt worried that I might have cancer as well. But I forgot about it soon. After my marriage (the couple have been married for four years), my husband told me one day "I had a dream your brothers came here and took away all your belongings". I suddenly thought to myself that I was about to die and my brothers would come over to get my stuff. I became so sensitive toward my dreams ever since, and because I really focused on my dreams, they became very real. The thoughts of death made me sensitive about myself, and I constantly had blood and urine tests and so on. Then it was my heart. I had electrocardiography which showed nothing. But I couldn't feel relaxed. Those who suffer from heart strokes have healthy hearts, but their heart suddenly stops beating, I told myself. That is why the tests weren't convincing to me. I thought about my body organs so much, that I was too

M. A. Besharat, *Paradoxical Psychotherapy: A Practitioner's Guide*,
University of Tehran Science and Humanities Series,
https://doi.org/10.1007/978-3-031-27717-7_14

aware of them. I was totally aware of my heart in my ribcage and I felt that a blow can make it stop beating. And now, I can't get my thoughts off my heart. It starts from the moment I wake till nighttime when I go to bed.

T: Well, the dream comes along and brings thoughts of death to your mind. Then, you gradually become concerned about your physical health and your body organs. Is that all, or has there been other symptoms as well (the usual symptoms of anxiety)?

C: Yes, there were severe anxiety, too. I went to a park close to our home, one day. I kept telling myself I was feeling dizzy so much that I actually began to feel dizzy. I thought I was about to die. I ran home an asked my husband to take me to a hospital. We went to a hospital and I had an electrocardiography, and the doctor said it was nothing serious and my pressure had dropped, probably. I never feel that my heart is heavy, doctor. It always feels light.

H: It also happened about her head too. She felt that her brain had become so small, or that she didn't have a brain, because her head felt so light.

T: (Addressing the wife) Is that right?

C: Yes, that's true. We were outside once, when I suddenly felt that my head was too light and I thought about my head so much that I forgot all about my heart. I kept thinking about my head (brain) for a couple of months before it got well and I went back to my heart.

T: Do you always have medical tests following such thoughts?

C: Yes, but the results of the tests, and the reassuring words of the doctors don't work on me.

H: Doctor, one of my wife's problems are the dreams she has. She has a dream about a magician who tells her she will never have a baby. She is really afraid and has decided that we should have a baby as soon as possible so that she can make sure that dream isn't true. Or she sees that it's the judgment day and the angels are asking questions from the dead. An angel says that her turn comes on Saturday. So, she keeps worrying that Saturday might actually be the day her dream comes true. The dreams happen again and again and she is mentally preoccupied with them. I just wanted to make her feel better, so I told her that her fears are probably due to eating certain types of food. As a result, she no longer eats fruits such as plums and strawberries because she thinks they don't agree with her. Or if we go to a party and it's meal time, she keeps asking whether the meat is lamb or beef, since she believes that beef doesn't agree with her. She has omitted a variety of food products from her diet so that she doesn't get worse. What I told her was not scientific, and I just wanted to make her feel better.

T: What other consequences have this problem had for you?

C: I feel like I have created a hell around myself. I think it's so easy to become crazy. I didn't have any problems, but I got myself into this mess through useless thoughts and fears.

H: Doctor, my wife's cousin is a great physician. We were at a party, and the cousin said that there is a blood vessel in the brain that can suddenly be blocked in young people and cause immediate death. We all heard and forgot it, but my wife couldn't forget about it ever again. She wanted to know more about brain vessels. She wanted to know whether it was possible for her to suffer from such a condition. Sometimes, she shows a blood vessel protruding out of her forehead saying "this means that blood can get to my brain." Later on, when she can no longer find the vessel, she says "what if there is a problem with the vessel and blood can't get to my brain?" Her whole attention is turned toward her body. All we talk about at home is health and different types of diseases. She keeps asking me to check her pulse and see if it's normal or not.

T: How long has it been since you had that dreams and the problems started?

C: It's been three years.

T: What about before that, before you got married? Did you have any similar experience then?

C: Before that, when I was a university student, I felt really worried when someone died and I couldn't stop thinking about it for several days. But I forgot all about it after a while. After I got married, it got worse. If I can go back in time, I will never let this happen to me, I keep telling myself. If I avoided these thoughts when they were just beginning, I would have been able to control them. Now, I can't get my mind off my body at all.

T: What have you done about your problem during the past three years?

C: I went through drug therapy (the husband points out that the drugs were Fluoxetine and Chlordiazepoxide) which made me a little bit better. But the problem came back.

T: Do you take drugs now?

C: No, I don't take any drugs at present.

H: We also went to a psychologist who taught her relaxation techniques, and I help her to do them at home. She does them some nights, but they don't work.

C: Doctor, now that we're telling you all this, I think how ridiculous this problem is, but I can't get rid of it nevertheless. I keep telling myself that God has created me and I can't have control over everything, but it doesn't work.

H: She says, sometimes, that she is afraid to go to sleep lest the dreams haunt her again.

C: I think that these thoughts come to me because I have nothing to do. Last year, we decided to have a baby so that I'd busy with the baby and don't have such thoughts. But I had to have an abortion, which made my body much weaker. I wanted to consult with you about pregnancy as well. Can I become pregnant under such circumstances?

T: We will talk about it later on. I need to know a little bit more. So far, I know that your mind is preoccupied with health and illnesses, the vital bodily functions and life and death. You also mentioned two more things. You (the husband) said that your wife doesn't come to certain parties, since she's afraid she might not have access to the hospital. And you (the wife) said that you were in a park and suddenly ran home and went to the hospital. Tell me more about this condition. You suddenly feel scared, and have to go to the hospital. Has this ever happened before? When did it first start? Let's consider this as a separate problem from the worries about your body. How can you describe it to me?

C: It was just those two times, and I don't remember anything else.

T: I will draw a timetable for you which you should do in order to get the best outcome. Now that you are receiving treatment under my care, it's better that you do not visit any other doctor or take any medication. Of course, you are free to do as you wish. However, if you want to follow the treatment here, you need to comply with this stipulation and not follow any other treatment procedure.

You are supposed to do a series of exercises according to the orders I give you. You position yourself in a quiet place, free from any distractions, for 10 min. You need to focus, and try to imagine and recreate all the thoughts and negative emotions about illnesses and your body organs, such as your brain and your heart. During the exercises, you must make an honest effort to remember all those thoughts about your body and feel the fear and the worry in all their intensity. Imagine that the blood vessel in your brain has been blocked and no blood can get to your brain and you are about to die. Your heart doesn't beat, and you are about to have a heart attack and then it will all be over. You must try to recreate and re-experience them as closely identical to the real experience as possible, within 10-min exercises. Several possibilities might present themselves. You do the exercise, and you manage to make it identical to the real thoughts and fears. We will get the best results if this happens. You may do your best during the exercise, but you can only manage to recreate the thoughts and fears by 50%, or you may fail to recreate them altogether: zero. It's okay for any of these to happen, as long as you make your best effort. There is also another possibility. You miss the exercise because you forget, or you don't find the appropriate place. If this happens, you simply skip that exercise and do not try to make up for it on another time. This is because you either do the exercises precisely on time, or you do not do them at all. Now, give me three times when you can do the exercises, starting from tomorrow.

C: But doctor, the thoughts and fears are always with me. I'm never free of them.

T: Good point. The thoughts occupy your mind 24 h a day. Is that right?

C: Yes.

T: You don't want them. They come regardless of what you want. However, during the three exercises, you actually want to have and experience them. You summon them and try to re-experience and relive them in your mind. The only difference is that while you don't want them at other times, you do want them during the exercises. Now, when can you do the exercises?

C: At 12:00, 17:00 and 22:00.

T: There are some other things you should know in order to be able to do the exercise correctly. First of all, start doing the exercise tomorrow. So, you don't do anything today. Second of all, you must do the exercises precisely on time. You can't do them any sooner or later than the time we have agreed on. If you cannot do any of the exercises on time for any reasons, skip that exercise and wait for the next one to show up. Thirdly, we agreed that you are about to do three 10-min exercises a day. It doesn't mean that you should try to avoid the thoughts and fears at other times of the day or that you should try to fight them in any way. You know you cannot avoid them in the first place. But what I mean is that you should not even make the effort in any way to prevent or decrease them. You do not decide nor desire to decrease them. Keep this in mind all through the treatment. You don't even do those relaxation exercises you told me about. Just do the three exercises, on time, according to my instructions.

(Addressing the husband) Now, you said that you talk a lot about body, health and illness. What else do you do?

H: I check her pulse, and I listen to her heart beat with a stethoscope. I interpret her dreams at times. Of course I make optimistic and positive interpretations all the time, and reassure her that her pulse and heart are working normally.

T: From now on, you don't do or say anything about her problem other than what I am about to tell you. You don't even have the right to remind her of her exercises or ask her questions about them. You don't interpret her dreams either. At present, you just check her pulse and her heart beat twice a day; before going to work and after coming back home. Both times, you must tell her "your pulse and heart are awful and you are done for." That is all you have to do. You can't do anything else, even if your wife asks you to. And you can't skip doing what I asked you to, even if your wife asks.[1] See you in two weeks.

Session Two

T: Welcome. Please tell me what you did.

C: I did the exercises, but I didn't quite realize why you said I should think about them voluntarily only within those three 10-min sessions. Because at other times, I sat down and thought about my body voluntarily.

T: Voluntarily, other than your home works?

C: Yes.

T: Willingly, or unwillingly?

C: Yes, I sit down and think, willingly, that my hart has become very small and is not working properly. I think that my brain has become small.

T: Are these thoughts worrying or pleasurable?

C: Of course I get worried.

T: Then they are not voluntary and willing. It is only voluntary when you can choose to do it if you like, and not to do it if you don't want to. If it's voluntary, and you see that it's painful to you, you can choose not to do it anymore. When you realize that fire burns your hand, you willingly choose not to touch it so that you don't get burned. These thoughts are involuntary, however. You hate them and don't want to have them, yet they come to you. These are all

[1] Taking into account the inevitable influence of the husband, as a member of the system, on her and her condition, couple therapy within the PTC model was taken into account from the beginning of the treatment. Later on, the value of the pathological interactions of the couple is removed and normal interactions take their places. The improvement made by the client allows her, in session six, to adopt a stance toward the husband that he has adopted toward her now. Pay attention to the final statements made in session six. You can see the switching of places between the wife and husband. These techniques and their effective mechanisms have been discussed in detail in *PTC perfect model of therapy with couples: A practical guide* (Besharat 2018).

involuntary. The only voluntary thoughts and fears are those you do during the 10-min exercises you accepted to do according to my orders.

C: But doctor, the exercises were no different from other times.

T: By what percentage did you manage to do the exercises?

C: I guess I did them by more than 90%.

H: I think the thoughts even increased, because she was given permission to think them.

C: No, they didn't increase.

T: (Addressing the husband) You were supposed to stay out of this and don't meddle in her treatment (the wife laughs). It is necessary that you follow my orders as well.

H: Of course.

T: This is because you may be part of the problem. You just do as I tell you. You were supposed to check her pulse during the two weeks. (Addressing the wife) What did he do?

C: He checked my pulse every morning, and told me that I was not in a good condition and maybe I will never see you again when I get back from work. And he did the same when he got back from work.

T: Did he do this regularly during the two weeks?

C: He did most of them.

T: And did you like him to do it?

C: Well, doctor, I knew that he was role-playing, so I didn't feel bad. Because it was fake.

T: What was the difference between these new check-ups and the old ones?

C: When he checked my heart and pulse according to your instruction and told me I wasn't healthy, I didn't feel bad. Before this, he said I was fine and reassured me. However, the ones he did according to your orders didn't make me feel anything.

T: Well, another issue we discussed the previous session, but for which I gave no orders, were your dreams. What happened to them during the last two weeks? Was there any change?

C: No, there was no change.

T: So, the dreams were the same.

C: I didn't have a dream that would upset me and make me think about it all the time. My dreams were normal.

T: So, why is it that you say there was no change? (Addressing the husband) Do you think the dreams were different?

H: I think they were. Before this, she always had bad dreams.

T: I asked this because I want you to pay close attention to your condition and make the right evaluation. If you have reported correctly that you have not had a bad dream during the two weeks, it means that change has taken place. Because, you must have had at least one bad dream. We should consider this change in bad dreams as a positive sign, unless the opposite of it happens in the future. Why is it that we should consider it a positive sign? Because something constructive has happened, and I have to rely on the report you give me today, so as give your next home works.

For the next two weeks, your exercise is the same as before according to my instructions. The only difference is that you must do the exercise every two hours, for 5 min. From the moment you start a new day, you do this 5-min exercise every two hours up to when you go to bed.[2]

(Addressing the husband) You no longer check your wife's pulse or ask her about how she feels. On odd days (determined through consulting the couple), you listen to your wife talk about her symptoms and bodily conditions such as her heart and brain for 15 min. In other words, you engage in the kind of conversation that you have always had. At other times of the day, you don't tell her anything, and if she wants to talk to you, you tell her "doctor has forbidden us to talk about that." When can you do the fifteen minutes?

H: At nights, when I'm home. 22:00 would be fine.

[2] This exercise is an example of increasing the dosage (the frequency of exercises). In cases when the paradoxical timetable cannot go its normal course of two to three sessions a day (the large number of the symptoms, the intensity of the symptoms, the chronicity of the condition, and the patient's characteristics), a solution is to break the barrier through increasing the number of exercises. As for this patient, the frequency of exercises increased to every hour which led to treatment outcome by 100%.

T: You can talk to each other for 15 min from 22:00 to 23:00. If you fail to do it within this time scope, you skip it and wait for the next day. Have a nice day, and see you in two weeks.

Session Three

T: It's nice to meet you again. Please tell me what you did.

C: I did the exercises, but I didn't get much better.

T: Well, tell me exactly what you did.

C: I did the exercises every two hours. However, the thoughts were still with me between the exercises.

T: The thoughts didn't leave, right?

C: Yes. Maybe last year, I could stop the thoughts from coming to me. But now, they overcome me completely and I can do nothing about them.

H: She has had dreams about death for consecutive nights. The dreams that had ceased for some time, have started again. She dreamed that she had lost her teeth. The last time she had such a dream, her grandmother died. And she believes that dreaming about losing your teeth means grief in life. The next night, she dreamed someone was reciting Quran on the player. She was really disturbed, so I told her "you can think about these dreams too, during the exercises."

T: You did the exercises every two hours, but the thoughts were still there. You said you didn't feel much better. What does that mean? Were there no progress at all?

C: There was. I felt a little better a couple of days ago, but I felt bad the next day again. Sometimes, I felt like I was all better, but then I got upset again.

T: So it is not like we can tell you have become better by 10–20%, is it?

C: Oh yes, I am better by about 10–20%.

T: Please pay attention that you said you felt better a number of times, but then the bad thoughts came back and overcame you again. This can be called some sort of change. But when you say that you've been better by 10–20%, it means that the better mood has been continued. Which one is it?

C: I was fine from the afternoon till night. After a number of daily exercises, I felt I was all better. But when I woke up the next day, it was all back.

T: Maybe if we talk about the interval between the exercises individually, you can have a closer estimation. For example, the interval between the first and the second exercise, the second and the third exercise, and so on.

C: When I woke up at 11, I felt bad. When I did the second exercise at 13, I was still feeling bad. But I felt good by 17. And when I felt all better when I was going to bed.

T: Do you wake up at 11 because you sleep late at night, or what?

C: No, I simply sleep a lot.

T: Good, and do you sleep well and does it refresh you?

C: Yes.

T: You do not take drugs, do you?

C: No.

T: Now, you said that you feel bad when you wake up in the morning. What do you mean by bad?

C: I feel weak when I wake up in the morning. I feel that I don't have any energy.

T: Some people say "it's difficult for me to get out of bed, I can't leave my bed, I don't have motivation…".

C: No, I'm not like that. I wake up easily. But my mind immediately goes to my body. I feel like my body is empty. Or, I think that my heart, which is a very important part of my body, has come to the surface of my body because I have thought about it so much, and it is therefore in danger. Or, I feel that my body is not solid enough to keep my heart safe.

T: Well, we know that these thoughts come and annoy you. However, what do you think about them? Do you consider such ideas right or wrong?

C: I can't say they are wrong. I think that my body is so weak that it has become empty, and so my heart is in danger.

H: A problem with her is that she is so negative. She is quite hopeless, asking "will I ever be healthy again?" Or, she says "I will never feel good again and the doctors will abandon me." She always sees the glass as half empty.

C: I am not always like that. I'm not like that in my life. I'm just like that when it comes to my problem and my physical weakness.

T: In my opinion, you have made good progress. You experience a lot of pressure and worry about your life, and disturbing thoughts do not let you to feel peace of mind unless you have made some definitive improvement. You are of course right, but I believe that you have made good improvement. You should keep in mind that improvement and treatment is gradual, and not sudden, and you should do your exercises patiently. There may even be regress through the process of treatment. There are times when after making progress by 40%, there is a regress by 10%. We have to move on, however, until we manage to overcome the problem completely.

Now, please tell me about the times we allocated for talking to one another.

H: We did them, in general. There was only one time when I was on a trip. Other than those times, on three occasions, she really insisted on talking. I asked her to wait till night when it's the time for talking.

T: How was it at other times?

H: She wanted to talk several times, but I stopped her and told her it can only be at times the doctor has assigned.

C: I did want to talk about it several times. But, in general, I feel that it has become less than before. I no longer need, as much as I used to, to talk about it with my husband.

T: As for the rest of your work, you need to do your daily exercises, starting from tomorrow, every hour for 5 min. At nights, when you want to go to bed, think to yourself, and actually wish, to have those disturbing dreams. As long as you are awake, you should consciously want to have those bad dreams. Keep on doing the conversation exercises on odd nights, for 15 min.

C: Doctor, we are going on Hajj next Monday.

T: That's quite all right. I will have another session with you next week, before you go.

Session Four

T: Welcome. Tell me what you did, and when are you going to Hajj?

C: We will leave tomorrow. I did all the exercises during the week, and I feel much better. But I feel I still need more time to get completely better.

T: Can you tell me in what ways you have improved?

C: Before this, the thoughts bothered me while watching TV. But last week, the thoughts weren't there while watching TV. I used to have the thoughts when I was busy with something. Last week, I didn't have them when I was busy. Another point is that when I wanted to think about those thoughts and bad moods during the exercises, I couldn't summon them at all.

T: This report shows that the process of treatment has started for you. But, as you mentioned yourself, it is not completed yet. You are like someone who has gone through surgery. She has been cured, and is getting better. But she is still recovering from her surgery and must be careful and take certain considerations into account. Today, I explain to you the considerations. At the same time, you are going on Hajj tomorrow. Any trip causes a certain level of stress, and under the present circumstances, it is not recommended. However, you must go on this journey.

How were your dreams during the week?

C: I did the exercises, doctor, but I had different dreams.

T: Were those dreams upsetting for you?

C: No, they were mainly unimportant dreams. Just once, I dreamed that a distant relative had passed away, but I didn't feel that bad because I did not know him well. If it was someone close to me, I would have felt horrible.

T: You must pay attention that through doing exercises (both the daily ones about worrying for your health, and the ones at night about your dreams) and welcoming them into your life, you have been able to decrease the pressure of the anxiety caused by the thoughts and worries. You were able to experience them consciously and willingly (and not unconsciously and unwillingly) as I'd asked you to do, and you saw the outcome. In other words, before this, they kept attacking you and you were worried and scared and didn't want to face them and deal with them. Through this method, you faced your fears and worries. You welcomed them and asked them to come to you. You faced them bravely and this made them go away. I want you to be aware of this.

(The husband had been trying to take care of and treat the wife during the conversation sessions. Therefore, the couple were given instructions to refrain from doing it anymore.) During your journey, you may not find much time to do the exercises. It is all right. If you find the chance, do the exercises, and if not, it's still okay. When you come back and the subsequent visits by your family are over, keep on doing the exercises of the previous session (both about the thoughts and the dreams) for two weeks. Then, it's our summer break and we will have no more sessions till September. I expect there will be no need for you to do any more exercises after the two weeks, and you can lead a normal life. If the thoughts come to you and keep bothering you again, you can draw a similar timetabled tasks and stick to it.

C: The thoughts and worries didn't come, no matter how hard I tried during the afternoon and the night exercises.

T: In such cases, when you do your best but the thoughts don't come to you, finish the exercise after one or two minutes. Whenever you can tell by experience that the thoughts will no longer come, you don't need to go through the 5 min.

C: Doctor, do you think I'm ready for pregnancy?

T: In my opinion, you had better wait till September when we have another session and I can see you again. Then, I can give you a final answer. Be patient.

Session Five

T: Welcome back. It's nice to see you again. Please tell me about yourself.

C: Thank you. Doctor, I didn't feel well during the journey. When we got back, I restarted the exercises and did them every hour, according to your assignments. In the end, I was really tired of the thoughts and didn't want to think about illnesses. I'm still not completely free of all bad thoughts, as I was years ago. But, I'm much better. It's not like I suffer from the thoughts all the time.

H: After we came back from Mecca, we didn't do the 15 min conversation exercises anymore. My wife thought that she didn't need them anymore. During the past two weeks, however, she asked me twice or three times, to check her pulse and pressure. She started her exercises quite well, but they became less and less frequent. For the past month, she didn't need to do them at all. In August, I took her to my work so that she wouldn't be lonely all the time.

T: So, you came back from Mecca. You did the individual exercises for some time and then you gave up. You didn't do the couple exercises, because you (the wife) didn't need them anymore. And you have started this job since August. You said that you felt good after the journey and the thoughts rarely happened. Can you give me a percentage?

C: I only have 30–40% to go (I'm better by 60–70%).

T: How about the dreams?

C: I do have dreams, but they are not disturbing ones. They are normal and unimportant dreams.

T: You are now like a runner who has ran for several kilometers and has reached the end. Yet, you cannot stop all of a sudden. You have to do exercises for several minutes that prepare your body for rest. Under the present circumstances, you mustn't omit the exercises. I said from the beginning that you must live with these thoughts for some time. Accept them for the present and let them be with you in the form of exercises. For now, get rid of the idea that there should be no disturbing thought. You must keep on doing the exercises twice a day, for 10 min. You can do them at work and at home. Tell me when you can do them.

C: Since we come home later from work, it's better that I do both at work, at 11:00 and 17:00.

T: And we need to define two 15-min exercises for conversation about the illnesses and health with your husband. Check something or let him check your pressure. But, pay attention that at other times during the day, you two are forbidden to talk about these matters. (Addressing the wife) You may really want it and not be able to leave asking for it, but your husband must not agree to do it. He can only cooperate with you during the two times we have agreed on.

C: We can do them Mondays and Thursdays at 23:00.

T: See you in two weeks.

Session Six

T: It is nice to see you. Please tell me what you did.

C: I did the exercises, but I didn't need the talk that much.

H: We were very busy at our institute during the last two weeks. She did her exercises during the day, but she didn't talk to me a lot. We did it only once or twice.

T: Why didn't you talk?

C: It was because I didn't suffer from those thoughts anymore, and I didn't have a problem that would upset me and make me want to speak to my husband about it.

T: How were you with respect to the thoughts?

C: I was much better.

H: Her complaints about her heart, brain and kidneys and the lightness of her head are over. But she talks about new things, at times.

T: Like what?

H: She said "I feel blood doesn't reach the hair on my head."

C: No, it was because my head was itchy and my hair has become so long, so I didn't feel well. But it's not like those worries.

T: (Addressing the husband) Did you mean that those worries are over, but something new—sensitivity toward hair—has taken their place?

H: Yes. Those thoughts and worries are over and I think that this new sensitivity about her hair has taken their place. I think that she still suffers from those worries, but she doesn't talk about them in order not to upset me.

C: No, no, it's not like that. Those thoughts aren't with me anymore. I would have told you if they were.

T: I am with you (the wife) on this point. Look! The nature of this problem is in a way that it cannot be kept hidden. If it's there, it makes some noise (the wife laughs). This is because the thoughts are so annoying that one who suffers from them cannot have peace of mind. It was just like that with you. You have both witnessed those thoughts and worries in the past, and you have both experienced the reactions they caused. Those tests, those visits to numerous doctors, the talks, the obsession with finding the right food, the dreams and all the disturbances were there and could not be denied. She could not act like they weren't there. If there are still with her now, they show some signs. I think you have reached a stage when we no longer need to have sessions. However, I still arrange one more session for you to do another check-up. Remember that you were the one who were able to deal with all those upsetting thoughts about your heart, brain, kidneys and so on. You were able to overcome your fears and remove them. It's been some time since you've been doing the exercises, and you have learned quite well how to do them. In the meantime, if the thoughts come back, or even if anything new happens, first wait for a couple of days. Let the thoughts be with you for five days. On the fifth day, draw a similar timetable for yourself and start doing the exercises. You can either have three 5-min exercises a day, or do the exercise every hour. You will get the same results. Just, don't be impatient. You don't need to act immediately, because there is the possibility that the thought goes away after a couple of days. If it doesn't, then you can start. We do the same thing in our daily lives. We don't think we have a cold the minute we sneeze. We don't immediately go to the doctor for any slight problem. We first hope that it's nothing important. We wait for it to go away. If it doesn't, then we think of a solution. This is what you need to do in this case. As for talking with your husband, if you feel that you can't keep it from your husband and need to talk to him about it, arrange another exercise for the conversation as well. Two 10-min exercises a week would be enough.

For the next two weeks, do the individual exercises once a day for 5 min (C: At 17:00); after that, do the individual exercises only on even days and do the couple exercise Friday nights, for 10 min.

As for the pregnancy, which you asked about, I don't think there is a problem. I think you are ready and you can do it. Is there anything else?

C: Doctor, there is a problem with my husband that has been really bothering me. My husband keeps plucking his eyebrows and eyelashes out. I think this is a problem. It's not normal and has been really bothering me (the husband start laughing). He laughs at it, but I don't like it. Sometimes, I feel that the bad thoughts come to me because I'm worried about him. (laughing) Doctor, please do something for him, as well.

H: It is because of our difficult business at work.

C: No, doctor. He was like this since the beginning of our marriage. Whenever he was deep in thought, he started pulling at his eyebrows. If I arrived a little late, I saw that he had pulled all his eyebrow hair strings out.

H: This habit goes back to when I was in high school. Every time I wanted to solve a mathematical problem, I fidgeted with my hair, which gradually turned into pulling at them.

T: (Addressing the husband,) in case you are willing, we can draw a timetable for you so that this habit goes away. (Addressing the wife,) thank you for mentioning it. However, in order for any psychological treatment to be successful, the person must want to help himself in the first place. If he is unwilling to deal with the problem, it cannot be solved.[3]

Session Seven

T: It's a pleasure to meet you again. Please, tell me how you have been.

C: Doctor, I feel I no longer need the exercises. Sometimes, although I remembered to do the exercise, I suddenly forgot about it. And when I sat down to do the exercise, I couldn't summon the thoughts at all.

T: How are you in general?

C: I'm quite fine. I'm just a little stressed about the baby (the husband confirms the recovery).

T: How long have you been pregnant?

C: I'm in my fourth month.

T: Great. A little stress about having a baby is quite normal. Everyone has that much stress, especially you who have undergone an abortion. But in my view, there cannot be a problem.

The therapist gives the client complementary explanations about how to prescribe the paradoxical timetable for herself with respect to worries about pregnancy and her baby. The husband was asked again to not interfere in the process. The possibility was discussed that his interference might be due to his own obsession, and it was decided that he needs to visit the doctor for treatment too, in case he cannot prevent his interferences. This is because he plays an important role as a family member.

[3] Personal determination and willingness to make changes and receive treatment are at the core of any type of psychotherapy. Adopting a decision to begin treatment can be caused by outer obligations or requests. However, before the process of treatment begins, the client needs inner motivation and obligation so as to be able to cooperate through the process of treatment. Refusal to accept one's problem and visiting a specialist can be due to any of the following reasons: ego-syntonicity of the disorder; the individual's personality characteristics; the values of the symptoms; the systemic and environmental requirements for the perpetuation of the disorder; chronicity of the disorder; the mean age of the patient and the disorder; and acceptance of the disorder.

14.3 Assessment of Treatment Outcome and Follow-Up

The course of the treatment was completed in 7 sessions. Assessment of the treatment outcome, which was based on the patients' comments in a graded scale of 0–100 and an open-ended question, indicated 90% recovery. A 34-month follow-up evaluation showed no relapse.

Client #13 (Male, 32 Years Old, Single)

15

15.1 Case Introduction

Mr. JM a 32-year-old single man came to the University of Tehran Clinic complaining about fears including fear of gonorrhea, syphilis, rabies and cancer starting years ago during his high school years. These fears continued till 6 years ago when they turned to fear of infection with HIV. Since then, JM started taking medicine mainly Fluoxetine and Sertraline with no improvement of his condition. The clinical interview based on DSM-5 (APA 2013), showed that JM had the criteria for illness anxiety disorder. JM's disorder had a great impact on his study, his job, and the relationships with people around him. This is his first time visiting for a psychological treatment rather than psychiatric medical-based treatment. JM was seen for 8 sessions over a period of 14 weeks.

15.2 Course of Treatment

Session One

Therapist (T): (After greetings, the initial talk and the social stage of the interview) Please tell me why you are here.

Client (C): I suffer from obsessive thoughts, which keeps bothering me. I'm taking medication now, so I'm better. But the moment I stop medication, it comes back. I've experienced it several times. My obsessive thoughts are about HIV. I'm afraid I might have it.

T: Since when have you had it?

C: I guess since years ago! I've had such obsessive thoughts since high school, but fear of HIV started six years ago. I was studying one morning, when suddenly it occurred to me that I might have HIV.

T: How were you before that?

C: I always obsessed over sexual issues. For example, if I had a fever blister, I thought that it may be gonorrhea or syphilis.

T: What else?

C: We live in a rural area. We used to have cats in our yard, and I kept thinking I might have cat rabies or something.

T: Okay. What else?

C: I was worried that I may get cancer and die.

T: So, you said that these worries and thoughts go back to your high school. Did you have any similar fears and worries before that?

C: Before that, someone slapped me in the face in a fight and I was really scared. A week after that, I had a seizure. I took Haloperidol for a year and I got well. I guess that might have caused all of it.

T: When did this fear, seizure and the subsequent medication occurred?

C: I was in the sixth grade.

T: And then, this condition continued up until the high school years, when it turned into the fear of gonorrhea, syphilis, rabies and cancer. Is that right?

M. A. Besharat, *Paradoxical Psychotherapy: A Practitioner's Guide*,
University of Tehran Science and Humanities Series,
https://doi.org/10.1007/978-3-031-27717-7_15

C: And then it was HIV. My sensitivity of HIV is horrible. I keep thinking that I may get it through sexual intercourse. This fear never left me alone up to now, which has been six years.

T: When did you start medication?

C: It's about six years.

T: Have you taken medication regularly since then?

C: It was regular, but I stopped it at some periods. When the obsessions came back, I restarted taking medication. I took Fluoxetine for a while. I stopped it for three months. When the symptoms reemerged, I took it again. I haven't taken many different drugs. It has mainly been Fluoxetine; and also Sertraline, for several months. Now, I take Fluoxetine, again.

T: How long have you been taking drugs non-stop?

C: It's been about two years now.

T: And you still have the obsessive thoughts?

C: They have decreased a lot, but they still keep bothering me. I've been feeling worse for some time now, and I know if I stop the medication, the horrible thoughts will haunt me again.

T: You have managed to quiet it down, but you know it's not gone away.

C: It won't go away. I'm sure it won't go away using drugs.

T: You're right. Drugs can't cure your problem. Now, tell me this: have you ever done anything about your problem other than visiting a psychiatrist?

C: I have been tested for HIV several times.

T: Have you done any tests about your former problems, such as cancer, rabies and gonorrhea?

C: No, I just did it for HIV. Every year (every other 12 months), I did the test, and it is always negative. I knew the tests weren't necessary, but at least they made me feel better. No sooner did I touch a public doorknob or something, when the fear of having contacted HIV came back to me again. I waited for a while before doing the test again, but I was restless and anxious. I have done the test five times so far. The last time was when I bandaged a student's injured hand in the football field. Suddenly, it occurred to me I might have contracted HIV through that student. In all these cases, I constantly check everything and try to convince myself through reasoning. I never touched his injured hand, I tell myself, and even if I did, my hand wasn't wounded in the first place. I keep giving myself reasons, and I feel convinced a little. After a while, though, the doubts come back and I simply have to do the test to make sure.

T: The reasoning doesn't work, and you give up and do the test at the end of the day. Is that right?

C: It turns into a vicious circle, and affects all my life and time.

T: Is there anything other than what you said so far? You mentioned that all the symptoms are sexual in a way. Why do you think so? Have you had any specific experience, problem or issue with respect to sex?

C: I haven't led a healthy sexual life. When I was a kid, we took the sheep to the plains for grazing. There were nobody around, there, and my cousins and I had sexual intercourse. We did it in turn. The intercourses didn't cause any problems for me. But, when officials started warning people of HIV in the country, I realized that HIV is contracted through sex, and the fears started. Years passed, I was the sexual partner to two different people at the same time. Then, I was studying one day when I suddenly asked myself, what if I have HIV?

T: So, these were the reasons you became more sensitive to HIV?

C: Yes. And I had a tendency toward homosexuality twice in my life. The first time, it was during high school when I was sexually attracted to a boy. And then, during the university years, I felt the same toward my roommate in the dormitory. They were girlish and so, I had sexual intercourse with them.

T: Does this mean that, in your sexual intercourse, you assumed the role of the male, while they assumed the role of the female?

C: It was reciprocal to some extent. But, mainly, yes. I usually assumed the role of the male. To be more precise: in the first relationship, I was more willing to assume the role of the female, while in the second relationship, I was more inclined toward being the male.

T: And how did you feel about the opposite sex?

C: I have never had a good relationship with the opposite sex. Before entering the university, I didn't talk to girls at all. And when I entered the university, I had no skills when it came to interacting with girls. I'm in a relationship with a girl at present, and we are thinking about marriage, but H have never been positive.

T: Do you have sexual desire for the opposite sex?

C: I do, but I like variety. I would like to experience being with numerous partners. Although, my religious beliefs have refrained me from doing so. But this is how I feel.

T: Have you ever had sexual intercourse with a member of the opposite sex?

C: I have, with the girl I told you about. We've been together for about two years and a half now. We haven't actually had sexual intercourse, but we have been together.

T: Why not?

C: There were times when I wanted it, but she didn't. So, I didn't insist a lot.

T: Did you feel satisfied?

C: Yes, we both reached orgasm.

T: Now, is your sexual preference mainly for the same sex or the opposite sex?

C: The opposite sex. I no longer have same-sex relations.

T: I need to explain to you two things, and then we make an arrangement for your present problem. Many people have had similar experience, especially in certain environments where it is more common. But, as you know, none of them, not even your cousin, have ever felt the problem that is bothering you. Is that right?

C: Yes.

T: It means that you have a certain level of sensitivity that has caused problems for you after the kind of experience you discussed. It's just like common cold that infects certain members of a family, but it doesn't necessarily infect all. The virus spreads to every member of the family, but the only person who gets the disease is the one who has certain characteristics. You have been ready, and sensitive enough, to feel such thoughts and worries. In other words, we can say that the thoughts and worries are not related to those experiences at all, as others who have had a similar experience haven't suffered from them.

Another point is that you must stop taking drugs today, as you did have the experience of stopping medication before. I will see you again in two weeks and we will start our treatment.

Session Two

T: We discussed your problem at the previous session, and you were supposed to stop medication, so that we can start our work in this session. Did you do it?

C: Yes, it's been ten days since I stopped my medication, and I have encountered no problems in this regard.

T: Thank you. What you will do as your treatment will prevent any possible side effects of ceasing your medication, if you do it right. Also, your fears and worries will be over forever. I first explain to you a unit of what you must do, and then I tell you when and how much you should do it. Each unit of your task is as follows: you go to a place where you can remain undisturbed, by people or the telephone, for 10 min. You must concentrate and try to remember and recreate all the annoying thoughts and worries about having HIV. Such remembering and recreating must be identical with the actual experience of having those worries and obsessions, and must be able to disturb you just as intensely. In other words, you are supposed to play the role of yourself suffering from the disturbing thoughts as artistically and precisely as possible. At other times during the day, the thoughts invade your mind without you wanting to have them. During these exercises, however, you summon the thoughts and worries about HIV and your declining health and recreate and re-experience them willingly, voluntarily and according to my orders. Several things might happen. You do the exercise honestly and seriously, take the bittern medication necessary for your health and manage to recreate the mood by 100%. We will get the best outcomes if this happens. If you can have an upsetting, disturbing experience within the 10 min, it's perfect. Despite your honest effort, you may only succeed to recreate the moods by 50%. This is still acceptable as long as you've done your best. There is also a third possibility. You try really hard, but the worries and fears cannot be recreated. There is zero similarity between the exercise and the real experience. Again, it's all right. The final possibility is that you don't do the exercise because you oversleep, you are not alone, you are outside home or you simply have forgotten all about it. In all such cases, the exercise is lost and you cannot make up for it at some other time. In other words, you either don't do the exercise, or you do it precisely on time. We arrange the times here for you. Starting from tomorrow, you have to do the exercises twice a day, each time for 10 min.[1] Now, if you have realized what you must do, give me two times during the day when you can do the exercises. You had better give me the times during which you are most likely to be able to do the exercises. At the same time, they should be as far away from one another as possible. We need two exercises a day for the first week, and one for the second week.

C: I have a very busy schedule. I don't think I can find any time.

T: Right now, the treatment of your problem must be your first priority. The right decision is to delay other programs in favor of doing this. You are now like an ill person who must be hospitalized according to the doctor's decision. Such a person are not even allowed to leave the hospital. He simply accepts the doctor's decision and is hospitalized. Such a person must cancel all his programs and appointments to do the surgery. You, however, don't have to cancel anything. You just have to consider the exercises as your priority during the two weeks. The first two weeks are absolutely important for a complete treatment.

C: 17:00 and 22:00 for the first week, and 22:00 for the second week.

T: There is something else in need to warn you about. When I told you to do the exercises at these specific times, it doesn't mean you must try to avoid or escape the fears and worries at other times. You have nothing to do with them at other times of the day. The obsessions might invade your mind unwillingly several times. But you have nothing to do with them. You must not try to prevent them from entering your mind. We will talk about whatever that happens in the next session.

[1] Due to the client's busy educational and occupational schedule, two instead of three exercises were defined for each day. Otherwise, the ideal combination consists of three exercises a day for the first week and two for the second week.

Session Three

T: Nice to meet you again. Please tell me what you did.

C: Doctor, I did the exercises regularly. But I was worried about my exams, so I didn't stop my mediation.

T: Well, the exams haven't allowed you to do according to our agreement. It's all right. We are close to our summer holidays, now. We can continue our treatment from September. Be sure to cease your medication two weeks before our next session together. Through the previous two sessions, I became familiar with your problem and you got to know my method. We can continue our work from September. In other words, the treatment begins in September (the fourth session). You can take medication as before, but you must definitely stop it two weeks before our next session.

Session Four

T: Nice to meet you. Following our preliminary sessions, you were supposed to stop medication so that we can begin our work. Tell me what you did and how you have been.

C: I didn't stop the medication until three days ago. I haven't taken medication ever since, but I know that it will all come back if I don't take drugs for two weeks.

T: What will come back?

C: Fear of having HIV. I am a teacher and I have to be in contact with students, to bandage their injuries and all that. This makes me think that I may have HIV. Of course, even if there are no such contacts, I still find other excuses to say that I may have HIV.

T: Well, what are the consequences of such thoughts and fears?

C: The consequence is constant tests. After the tests, I feel reassured for a week. But the thoughts come flooding back to me, and I am disturbed again. All these are accompanied with continuous mental reasoning. I keep using the fact to convince myself it's nothing. But it doesn't work.

T: You said that you have no doubt that drugs cannot help you.

C: Yes.

T: Drugs have caused you harm in yet another way. It has made you believe you can never quit it, even when you are receiving another treatment. It has made you certain that if you don't take it, you are sick. This is all the medication can do. It divests you of who you are and your abilities. Right now, you can't even tell yourself "what the hell, let's stop taking the medication under the supervision of another specialist and through using another treatment. What could happen? The worst case is that I will again be the sick person I've always been. And I can always begin using drugs again." Taking medication for several years have deprived you of the necessary motivation and the courage, and it prevents you from thinking correctly. The correct thinking here is telling yourself "all right, I won't take drugs for two weeks; and I'm going through another treatment within the two weeks. The worst case scenario is that the problem comes back after two weeks, and I will take medication again. I have already stopped medication several times."

I hope you can keep away from drugs for two weeks, this time. (Explanations similar to those of the second session were offered by the therapist). It was decided that the client must do two 10-min exercises during the first week, and three 5-min exercises for the second week. Taking into account the patient's ineffective coping methods, he was told not to look for reasons to convince himself that he does not have a disease. The client was asked to let go of this ineffective method.[2] You've been doing it for six years, all to no avail, and it's curious that you still won't let go of it (as you won't let go of useless medication). Quite the contrary, you must recreate and re-experience your fears in a way so as to think that you have really contracted HIV. You have to feel it so strongly that you are scared to your very soul. Even if you are dying of the fear of having HIV, you must neither make arguments nor take medication. You must only think that you have HIV. At what time can you do the exercises?

C: 17:00 and 22:00 for the first week, and 17:00, 20:00 and 23:00 for the second week.

T: You must also be careful not to try to fight the thoughts at other times of the day. You must do as a completely passive person who cannot make any decisions or help himself.

C: You mean that I shouldn't fight with the thoughts if they come to me at other times during the day?

T: You mustn't do anything about them at all. You will neither take drugs, nor make arguments or anything. You've been doing them for six years and you've gotten nowhere. Do as I tell you for some time and let's see what happens.

Session Five

T: Welcome back. Please, tell me what you did.

C: I did all but two of the exercises. But I couldn't recreate and imagine those thoughts in my mind, no matter how I tried. I think the effects of the drugs are still with me and don't let the thoughts to come alive and cause anxiety in me.

T: You have stopped your medication, haven't you?

C: Yes, I don't take them anymore.

T: What else?

C: That is all.

T: How were you at other times of the day?

C: I was fine. I didn't suffer from those thoughts anymore.

[2] As we said, in the PTC model, the patient is asked to give up all other personal and professional (drug therapy, parallel psychological interventions, etc.) solutions. One reason is that they function as barriers against the occurring the goals of paradoxical timetables. One manner of personal intervention includes coming up with attempts to rationalize the condition and its symptoms. The present client resorts to this method abundantly.

T: All right, we don't care right now why you weren't able to recreate the thoughts. Or why the effects of the medication is or isn't still there despite your prediction. The important thing is for you to stick to my instruction. Continue doing the exercises twice a day till the next session. Tell me the times.

C: 18:00 and 22:00.

T: Do the exercises for 5 min at these times. See you next session.

Session Six

T: Welcome back. Tell me what you did during the last two weeks.

C: I did the exercises according to the timetable, but I guess the thoughts made my mind more active. Because I had the thoughts about illnesses at other times. I think that the effects of the medication are wearing off and I know that when they are finally gone, the thoughts will come back. I'm sure the thoughts will not let go of me.

T: You said that the thoughts became active after some of the exercises. How long did they last?

C: They were with me for thirty minutes after the exercise. Then they went away.

T: You are completely sure that your illness will come back and will never leave, if you don't take medication again, is that right?

C: Yes.

T: It's been a month since you stopped taking the medication. Yet you keep believing that the thoughts haven't come back because of the drugs. Is that right?

C: Yes.

T: I hope you can manage to continue keeping away from the drugs. Do the rest of the exercises this way: our next session will be held in four weeks, due to the holidays. For the first two of these four weeks, do the exercises three times a day, each time for 10 min. For the second two weeks, do three 10-min exercises on odd days (agreed upon by the client).

C: I can do them at 14:00, 18:00 and 22:00.

T: You will do the exercises according to the instructions I gave you in previous sessions. You have been practicing with the thought of catching HIV. I want you to add another thought: imagine that you have ceased medication and the symptoms have come back. Imagine that the illness has come back.

Session Seven

T: Welcome back. Please, tell me what you did.

C: Doctor, I did the exercises. During the exercise, I let the thought come to my mind. I even managed to experience negative affects. But, there was nothing after the exercises. During the last week, something weird occurred to me. I felt a strange calmness after the exercises. It's been more than two months since I stopped my medication, and I can't understand why the thoughts have not come back yet.

T: Look! When you had stopped your medication for only three days, you were worried that the symptoms may come back after two weeks. After the two weeks, you said that the drugs are still effective. It's been four months now, and there are no symptoms. Yet you are surprised. You can't think for one second that maybe the treatment you are receiving, and the exercises you do, have helped you get over your condition. It's partly due to the fact that the medication has rendered you powerless, and partly due to other reasons which we cannot discuss here. Although you've been in a good condition for two months without needing to take drugs, your helplessness doesn't allow you to see the reality. You still need more time.

Your next task is to not follow any of the previous home works and do any of my exercises up until the next session, which is in two months.[3]

Session Eight

T: Well, it's been two months. Tell me how you have been.

C: After our last session, I didn't do the exercises for two weeks. After the two weeks, the thoughts were beginning to come back when I

[3] This task is a paradoxical one in its nature. It gives the patient the opportunity to do an experiment as he wishes. The report given by the patient in the next session shows the results of the experiment.

started doing the exercises again. The thoughts went away immediately.

T: How long did it take for the thoughts to go away again?

C: Within a week; this time, I believed that I was better as a result of doing the exercises, not taking the medication.

T: You are still not taking medication?

C: Yes, I haven't taken any medication ever since.

T: Well, you found the opportunity to stop the exercises once, feel bad again, restart doing the exercises and feel better. You did an experiment on yourself, and you found out about the outcome. Can you tell me in percentage terms how better you are?

C: I'm better by more than 90%, and the 10% belongs to thoughts that just come and go, and I know they are nothing serious.

15.3 Assessment of Treatment Outcome and Follow-Up

The course of the treatment was completed in 8 sessions. Assessment of the treatment outcome, which was based on the patients' comments in a graded scale of 0–100 and an open-ended question, indicated 90% recovery. A two-year follow-up evaluation revealed that there was no relapse.

16 Client #14 (Female, 62 Years Old, Married)

16.1 Case Introduction

Mrs. MK, 62 years old, was referred to the University of Tehran Clinic because of her anxiety attacks started at 25 along with nausea, spasm in the neck and jaw muscles. She had visited a psychiatrist and had received medication for 15 years. She ceased taking medicines 10 years ago, following which the physiological symptoms disappeared. However, the patient developed her new fears that she might, at any moment, have spasm in her neck and jaw muscles. She had severe religious guilt due to the fact that she had done things that were against her religious beliefs in the past. She had serious compulsions with checking the gas valve, door locks and the power button on TV. The anxiety symptoms included checking the possibility of breast cancer daily; extreme fear of getting blood cancer; extreme anxiety over her children's health and the fear that they may get cancer. The symptoms of compulsions and illness anxiety disorder with respect to her children started 6 years ago. Her symptoms fulfilled the DSM-5 (APA 2013) criteria for OCD and illness anxiety disorder. MK started taking medications again four years ago. At the time of visiting the therapist, she took 10 mg/day Fluoxetine. This is her first visit to receive a psychological treatment. MK was seen for 4 sessions over a period of 7 weeks.

16.2 Course of Treatment

Session One

Therapist (T): (After greetings and the social stage of the interview) tell me a little bit about what brings you here today.

Client (C): My problem started 25 years ago when my husband got married again (I had a 1.5 year-old daughter). This problem has been with me ever since and when I got angry, I felt nauseous and when I went to see a doctor, he would usually say I had food poisoning but there was no such thing as food poisoning. Later, the psychiatrist prescribed Diazepam and told me to inject a small dose into my muscle whenever I felt nauseous. Later on he asked me to have an intravascular injection which was supposed to help me sleep better, relax my body and improve my condition. When I threw up, my jaw deviated and my neck and mouth became stiff. After ten years, another doctor told me to stop doing the injections. He believed that this injection made my neck and mouth ache more. I no longer had a shot. I haven't had the jaw deviation for ten years. When I get angry, I feel nauseous and I throw up. I feel as if I'm dying. Although I haven't had neck and jaw cramps for ten years, I always feel I'll have one.

T: You mean you haven't had those cramps for ten years but you feel you will experience one, right?

M. A. Besharat, *Paradoxical Psychotherapy: A Practitioner's Guide*,
University of Tehran Science and Humanities Series,
https://doi.org/10.1007/978-3-031-27717-7_16

C: My daughter says I've been conditioned. Later, I visited a psychiatrist and I'd taken Fluoxetine for four years, which only increased my heartbeat and made me sleep 24 h a day, unfortunately. It's been three months since I stopped taking it. For ten years I had been struggling with this condition but for the last 7 or 8 months, it's been awfully hurting me. I've had obsessions; when one of the children leaves her lab test result at home, I always check to find out whether or not she has got a disease. This automatically happens to me. I feel guilty very much and I don't know what to do to erase all these from my mind. When I was young, I used to struggle with so many issues and now it's been 20 years since I gave up saying my prayers but I constantly think about the afterlife. What should I do to alleviate myself? How can I clean my mind? I feel like hell.

T: You said you have been suffering from this condition for the last 7 or 8 months. Does nausea bother you so much?

C: No it doesn't. Nausea has always been with me. For example, if I call my daughter right now and find out she is not well, I'll feel nauseous.

T: You feel nauseous?

C: Yes I do.

T: Is it only similar to nausea, or does nausea actually happen?

C: When I get a shot, I don't feel nauseous and have no negative feelings but if I don't, I feel terrible; the calcium in my blood drops; my hands were once paralyzed and the doctor said the calcium in my blood reached zero and so gave me a calcium shot in the volume expander and then I felt well. My children let the doctor know that I was not poisoned, and that my stomach had no problems whatsoever. They told him I felt the same way whenever I got angry.

T: Oh! So when you said it got worse in the last 7 or 8 month, you meant this. Right?

C: Yes. I get better once in a while but it gets worse at nights. I don't feel well, doctor.

T: Does it start with these thoughts?

C: Yes. I don't feel well at all, doctor. In all these conditions, feeling of guilt hurts me the most. I don't know what to do. I'm just struggling with God and myself.

T: What are your obsessions and/or compulsions about?

C: I have too much checking. For example, I sometimes turn the TV on and off several times. I constantly check the oven. I sleep and wake up during the night to check whether or not I've locked the door. I check and find out it is locked. Sometimes it becomes severe and at other times it does not and in those times, I become more relaxed. I've been both the father and the mother to my children. If my children are around, I feel better but generally I keep to myself; I feel depressed; I like to sleep a lot; I don't like to speak; Nothing seems new to me, doctor; I like to set my soul free, doctor. I don't know what to do. I wonder whether or not my mind will be clean if I get an ECT. Will that help me get rid of this suffering?

T: No. that's not the right way. Now that you've come, we will make a treatment plan for you and hope you succeed. So, you were talking about checking. Is there anything else?

C: I check myself 24 h a day. Because I am old, the doctor told me to take a Pap Smear every three months and check my breasts to see whether or not there's anything wrong. I check them 10 times a day. I ask myself why this part of my body is swollen. I must have a cancerous tumor. Why do I have anemia? I must have cancer. Because I have anemia, the doctor has given me iron tablets. I tell myself I must have blood cancer. You can't imagine how much I suffer, doctor!

T: When did all this start?

C: It's been with me for at least 5–6 years.

T: Are all these thoughts and doubts about cancer limited to personal inspection of your body, or have you had medical examinations as well?

C: I went to the doctor to get a mammogram and he said I was ok; I can't constantly go there and ask them to examine me.

T: So you just check to see whether or not those thoughts come to your mind.

C: Yes.

T: So let's recap: the feelings of nausea take place either when you get angry or when the negative thoughts come to your mind. And you have other obsessions about your own health and checking the oven, the door lock and television…

C: I also have obsessions about my children.

T: What do you mean by that?

C: I'm worried about my children's health conditions. I always think about their health and diseases. Last week, I went to get a sonogram with my daughter who is with me right now. I sat behind the veil and heard the doctor say my daughter had cancer. I had shivers down my spine, doctor. I felt terrible. I went in. The doctor was standing there. I asked what my daughter's problem was. The doctor asked why I went in. Then he wrote the examination result on a piece of paper and told me to read it. He said he was responsible to tell me the truth. I am sure I had heard him say she had cancer. I didn't tell her, but I told my elder daughter about it and she said if it were true, the doctor was supposed to give me the right answer. She read the paper the doctor had given me. The paper said she had a cyst and that its type was common. Everything seemed to be ok. That's all. But doctor, I heard him say she had cancer.

T: What else? What about washing and taking a bath?

C: No I don't wash a lot.

T: You said about your guilty feeling. How does this feeling of guilt manifest itself?

C: I regret what I did when I was young. When my ex-husband and I lived together, he would take me to the officers' club. He was a guard officer at that time and asked me to take off my veil whenever we attended those clubs. He believed it would have been insulting to others if I didn't. He asked me to drink and dance. He asked me to partner his colleague and he partnered his colleague's wife. This was a must in life in those days. Although I lived with him for 26 years, I was not able to continue it any longer because my family was religious; I committed a lot of sins.

T: Do you feel guilty for them?

C: My sister tells me to start saying my prayers again. I believe it's not possible to compensate for 30 years of prayers and fasting. I tell my children to avoid doing things that can make them feel guilty later in life. Always try to lead a healthy life. My children believe I've always been a good mother for them and have tried my hardest to be a good mother. I think I should not have done so many things I did. Those things bother me so much, doctor.

T: What pills do you take?

C: Just Fluoxetine; I take one Fluoxetine 10 mg a day. If I don't take it, nothing will happen.

T: Why do you take it then?

C: Four years ago, one of the doctors, who was close to me, told me to take one Fluoxetine a day.

T: You just said if you don't take it, there'll be no problem. Have you tried to stop taking it?

C: Yes. I didn't take the pills for a couple of months.

T: All right. Now after all these years, it's my turn to make a treatment plan for you. It will be a simple and special treatment plan that you can do to hopefully get rid of these problems. Let me explain something first. There are many people who might have done wrong and sinful deeds which they regret doing later in life. The person who has no mental problems and is normal knows what to do. She repents and does everything she can, such as saying compensatory prayers, to make up for her mistakes and when she honestly does so, she no longer commits the sinful deeds and she no longer considers herself a sinful person and keeps on living her life decently. That you were not able to do so stems from your problem. Do you know what I mean? If you didn't have this problem, you might try to compensate for your past by repenting. This applies to all people and when they reach this point, they feel better. They would say "Thank God we are informed. That thing happened and awakened us and let us recreate our life and afterlife." This makes them happy; they don't get sad. This sadness which exists within you is related to your problem. I want you to know it and don't confuse and mistake it with your problem. These are two separate issues. But what is this problem? What should we do about it? You are often at home, right?

C: Yes.

T: This is good because you will have enough time to do my treatment plan. In fact, all that is happening to you such as the checking, the negative thoughts and the feeling of nausea haunt you 24 h a day, bother you and you don't like them but they won't stop. You are stuck in this situation.

I will make some simple treatment tasks which you should carefully stick to. These tasks are like taking drugs and should be done carefully. One of the tasks is about the compulsive checking. Your task is to repeat checking the oven, the television and the door locks in a 6-min occasion, just as you do in your daily life. You should turn the TV on and off several times. Do the same for the oven and the door locks for 6 min. You should do the tasks three times a day and you ought to allocate 6 min to each task. The checking should be exactly similar to how you do it in your daily life. The only difference is that in your real life, these compulsive behaviors come to you unintentionally but here you do them of your own volition, but according to my instructions. You will start these tasks from tomorrow. Now give me three points during the day when you can do the tasks from tomorrow.

C: 12:00, 16:00, and 22:00.

T: There are two other points regarding the tasks which you should be careful about. You should do the tasks exactly on time, not before or after it. In other words, these tasks are either done on time or never done at all. If you happen to miss them on their proper time, you should skip them and you ought not to make up for them. There are times when you forget to do the tasks, or maybe you're not home, or have a guest. In any of these circumstances, you should skip the task without making up for it. Another important issue is that you are now responsible for doing these three tasks in their due time. This is all I ask you and you shouldn't do anything else about your problem. When I say you should check things on these three occasions, I don't mean that you should not check things at other times. Let the real checking come and go. You don't have to stop it. Do them whenever you feel the need. If the real thoughts come to you 10 times a day, act upon them; but do these three occasions for me too. That's all.

Your next task is to stay in a comfortable place according to the plan we will shortly make. Try to find a quiet place where you can focus and think about the issues I tell you. At these times, you are supposed to relive, recreate and review the thoughts about your past deeds, and the thoughts about the health and sickness of your children like the times when they automatically come to your mind. Try to recreate the negative thoughts and worries within yourself and try your hardest to suffer from them. Try to suffer just the way you explained to me. This task should last 5–7 min. Allocate half of the time to your past deeds and half to the health and sickness. This task is a little bit different from the first one. In the first task, you should have done a practical task which was quite easy. You simply opened and closed the door but here you should recreate the thoughts. There are some possibilities that can take place in the process of recreation and concentration. One possibility is that you concentrate on your past deeds and the sickness of your children and, as a result, you get annoyed and suffer from the condition. If that happens, it means that this intentional task becomes exactly like the real automatic thoughts, which will be wonderful and you will get the best results. This resembles a surgical operation which is difficult for the patient (now imagine that the patient is not conscious and has to suffer from so much pain) but after tolerating a little pain, his/her sickness will be treated. You are supposed to do such a task. In this task, you are your own surgeon and you are supposed to make an operation on yourself to get rid of your problem. However, there are times when you try your best but you are not able to achieve the desirable results. For instance, you try your hardest to get the results by 100% just like the real thoughts and feelings, but it doesn't happen; and only 50% of the expected result is achieved. If this happens, there will be no problem because you have done your duty. Even there are times when you try your best but you can't bring the thoughts to your mind at all. Nothing. There is no problem here either because you have done your job. Another possibility is the time when you happen to be asleep or someone is around. In this case, you are not able to do the tasks on their due time, and what you should do is to skip the tasks without making up for them. Now, what time is good for you?

C: 11:00 and 17:00.

T: All right. I need to mention a very important point here. Pay attention carefully. You just need to recreate the thoughts in these tasks. You are not allowed to stop these thoughts at other times. Let these thoughts come and haunt you just like the last thirty years. Don't do anything with them. Let them be repeated in your mind as much as they are supposed to. You are only supposed to do these two tasks I have told you and you should not do anything else.

C: Okay, doctor.

T: All these tasks will start tomorrow. Don't do anything today. Prepare yourself to do the tasks tomorrow. See you next session.

Session Two

C: Hello doctor.

T: Hello. It's nice to see you. Tell me what you have done so far. Did you do the tasks?

C: I did the tasks which were about the door locks, television and oven on two occasions but when I decided to do them on the third occasion, I thought it would be crazy to do so. I did the tasks only on two occasions and I criticized myself and said this would be meaningless to do these tasks three times a day. I said to myself that a sane person would not do that. Then I stopped doing that.

T: You stopped doing that. So you didn't do them?

C: No I didn't do them at all. For example, this morning when I was coming here, I locked the door but I didn't look back to check whether it was locked as I always did.

T: You didn't look back to check the door?

C: I said to myself when I locked the door, it would definitely be locked and there is no need to check again.

T: Good.

C: I did all the other tasks except for two of them. I forgot to do one of the tasks and missed the other one because I overslept.

T: Very well.

C: I did the tasks on two occasions having that kind of feeling but the rest was normal. The second time when I did the task, I had a headache. I saw myself in the mirror and I felt my face was bloated but after doing those tasks, everything went very well.

T: You mean you did the tasks but you felt normal.

C: Yes. The rest seemed normal and I felt better.

T: All right. You have had a good start and so far you have done great. Now, let's get ready to move on. We intentionally decided on a one-week period to test it and the beginning has been good. From now on, I'll see you every other week. Let me ask you one more time. You did the tasks on one or two occasions and then you felt there was no need to do so. Is that right?

C: Yes.

T: Did you feel there was no need at all?

C: Yes.

T: What did you feel was happening?

C: I thought to myself, this is not even what a sane person would do, and I stopped doing them.

T: In the past you felt the need to do so but now you don't feel this compulsion.

C: I don't feel the need to do anything at 16:00, 12:00, and 22:00.

T: Didn't you feel the compulsions at other times? Were you comfortable?

C: I have been fine this week, doctor.

T: All right.

C: Last time when I saw you, I was mentally wrecked doctor, I was not comfortable at all and didn't have the faintest idea how to free my mind but I've got better this week. I feel more comfortable.

T: All right. This time, do the tasks for three days. Today, tomorrow and the day after tomorrow. Do the checking as I instructed you. What time were you supposed to do them? Do you remember?

C: At 12:00, 16:00, and 22:00.

T: You should do the tasks at 12:00, 16:00, and 22:00 today, tomorrow and the day after tomorrow.

C: Thank you doctor.

T: Regarding the second task, you should continue doing the tasks about your past and the health and sickness of your children for another week. Do them thoroughly twice a day. What time do you prefer to do them at?

C: At 17:00 and 23:00.

T: Do this task at 17:00 and 23:00 for a week for five minutes. After the second week, you just need to do them once. I want you to do another task on two occasions. Your new task will last ten minutes. During the first five minutes you should think about cancer or any other diseases that you already thought about and try to make your feelings be as real as possible. For the second five minutes, you should look at yourself in the mirror. You should check yourself and during this task, be sure that you are inflicted with a deadly disease and imagine that your death is near. Just like the previous tasks, do the tasks about the sickness, and checking willingly according to my instruction. Let's see when you can do them on the third week. You will do the previous task within five minutes and you also need two occasions, 10 min each, for the new task. So what will it be?

C: 12:00, 16:00, and 22:00.

T: 12:00 is supposed to be for continuing the previous exercise and 16:00 and 22:00 are for the new task. Have you taken pills?

C: I no longer take Fluoxetine.

T: Never take any more pills and keep in mind never to do anything more apart from the tasks themselves. Do these tasks till the next session.

Session Three

T: It is nice to see you.

C: Thank you doctor. Thanks a million for taking the time to see me. Let me say first that I've not done all my homeworks. Since last week, I've had a guest and so I was not able to do the tasks for three days.

T: No problem. It's normal. Let's see how much you've done in general. We decided that the checking should continue a little bit and be put an end to. Also, we agreed that the thinking about the problems of the children and yourself should continue too. How much of all these have you done?

C: I've come to visit you about three sessions which lasted four weeks. Doctor, I used to say prayers, struggle with my conscientious and do whatever I could to solve my problems with no success, but for the last twenty days, I've no longer thought about those issues and I feel content about my condition. I used to go around the house and check the telephone, the oven and things like that but I don't do them anymore. Regarding the task about my sickness and checking myself, I did it for a couple of times but it got boring and I no longer did it because I had no more feelings about it. I felt more comfortable about my past too.

T: What about your problem about the sickness of your children?

C: I've been better. I was able to be stay away from my children and call them fewer. I used to be more curious about them but I'm no longer like that.

T: In previous session, I asked you to focus more on yourself, on your sickness, and on checking and examining yourself. How was everything?

C: Doctor, just let me do the plan for another week because I was not able to do this task well enough.

T: We will get to that, but I'd like you to give me an account of how you have been during the last week.

C: I've been better but I'm worried about feeling nauseous again.

T: We've not get to that. We will put it on the agenda, but not yet. We will deal with that soon.

C: Thank you so much doctor. I've been able to live a different life during this period.

T: Look! We have three weeks till the next session. During these three weeks, start doing the two tasks tomorrow for three days. On one occasion, recreate the thought about the children's sickness and on another recreate the thoughts of your own sickness, each for five minutes. Do them according to the instruction I already gave (C: The thought about the children, at 17:00 and the thought of myself at 23:00). After three days, just review and recreate your own thoughts and the task about the sickness of your children will be finished (C: My own task will be at 23:00). From the second week, you will have two tasks, each of which will last for five minutes. Recreate the thought of your own sickness on one occasion and examine and check yourself on another (I'll recreate the thought of sickness at 17:00 and I'll examine and check myself at 23:00). The task of the third week is very important and has to be done carefully (C: I'll do them at 17:00 and 23:00).

Session Four

C: Sorry, I had to change the time of my previous appointment.

T: No problem. It's not so bad because now that we are seeing each other, such a long time has passed. How's everything been with you?

C: I've got much better doctor. I'm very well. Occasionally, I thought the freckle on my neck was due to some serious disease, but I instantly said to myself it isn't anything special. It's just like a wind which blows and goes away. But generally, I'm fine. I owe you very much.

T: You're welcome. Thanks God. I'm glad that you feel better. I'd like to know about the last task I asked you to do. What happened to the feeling of nausea and the deviation of your jaw?

C: I did that too but I'd like to do this task for one more week.

T: What have you been feeling during these four weeks, especially the last two weeks?

C: I feel better. In the past, I asked everyone not to look at me wherever I went because I was afraid that my jaw would deviate but I didn't feel like this during this period.

T: How about other things? What about the feeling of guilt, and the sickness of your children?

C: Regarding the feeling of guilt, I always thought I would not be able to compensate for my past and I always had the negative feelings about myself and the afterlife within me. Hopefully, I don't have those feelings. I feel comfortable and I can easily say my prayers. Regarding the sickness of my children, I stayed away from them and I no longer asked or called them and when we speak, I don't ask about these issues anymore.

T: Are you still worried that your jaw might be deviated?

C: No I'm no longer worried about that.

T: How have you been feeling during the last month?

C: I have been feeling really well. My life has changed. I am relieved. I've found the comfort in life. I'm living quite well with your help, doctor. Thank you so much.

T: You have done a great job so far and you are well now. I'll make a two-week treatment plan for you so that you can continue to do them during the New Year's Holidays. If you feel the need for seeing me, you can make an arrangement but I don't think it will be necessary. Repeat the last tasks for the next two weeks; the feeling of nausea and the deviation of your neck. Do the tasks twice a day during the first week and allocate ten minutes to each task (C: 24:00). Allocate half of the task to the thought of sickness, examination and getting the nausea feeling and allocate the other half to the cramps in the neck. I hope you won't need to come here again but if you do, I'll be available.

C: Thanks a million. I'm so grateful.

16.3 Assessment of Treatment Outcome and Follow-Up

The course of the treatment was completed in 4 sessions. Assessment of the treatment outcome, which was based on the patients' comments in a graded scale of 0–100 and an open-ended question, indicated 100% recovery. A 22-month follow-up evaluation showed no relapse.

17 Client #15 (Female, 35 Years Old, Married)

17.1 Case Introduction

Mrs. MM a 35-year-old married woman came to the University of Tehran Clinic complaining about serious fear and anxiety attacks, compulsive checking and cleaning, irritability, and depressive mood. She described her present state as “things have lost their values in my eyes. I don’t care if it’s my husband, mom or dad. I don’t like this life any more”. MM reported a history of having compulsive cleaning and washing during her childhood. She described herself as a very brave person having no fears at all until one or two months ago that all fears and anxieties started. MM was first referred to a psychiatrist and took medication for a short period till a week before her first session of psychotherapy began. Her symptoms fulfilled the DSM-5 (APA 2013) criteria for panic attack disorder accompanied by symptoms of depressive disorder. MM is living with her husband and their only child and this is her first visit for psychological treatment. MM was seen for 3 sessions over a period of 4 weeks.

17.2 Course of Treatment

Session One

Therapist (T): (After greetings and the social stage of the interview) Please tell me why you are here.

Client (C): I wasn’t even afraid of the Grim Reaper before. But it’s been a month now that a weird fear has gripped me. I cannot go out at nights. I am afraid of the dark. If there is scary movie on TV, I can’t watch. If I see a disabled or sick person somewhere, I get scared. I wasn’t scared of anything at all. My husband worked at the night shifts for a whole year, and I spent the night with my little baby all alone. And I wasn’t afraid at all. Nowadays, when he goes to work at 4 am, I get so scared that I can’t go back to sleep until sunrise.

T: What scared you this much all of a sudden? What happened?

C: It was at night time. We had guests over. When they wanted to leave, I saw there were a crowd of people on the street. I asked my husband to go and see what’s wrong. He came back and said that a drug-addicted man had overdosed and was lying unconscious on the street. Then we got in the car to give our guests a ride home. My body started shaking and it was totally out of my control. They kept telling me I shouldn’t be afraid, but it was useless. The fear has been with me ever since. I trembled for a whole week. Now that I’m recounting it, I am scared. I was scared out of my wits. For the first week, my husband waited for the sun to rise so he could leave for work. I said prayers and recited holy Quran, but it didn’t help. I was gradually getting better. However, two weeks ago my husband came home and said that he had seen another drug-addicted man in the alley, and had sent him

M. A. Besharat, *Paradoxical Psychotherapy: A Practitioner’s Guide*, University of Tehran Science and Humanities Series, https://doi.org/10.1007/978-3-031-27717-7_17

away. But it made me scared again. I have a fast heartbeat, I can't go anywhere at nights, and things have lost their values in my eyes. I don't care if it's my husband, mom or dad. I don't like this life any more. My husband takes me out so that I can feel better, but it's useless. I spent some time with my parents who live in another city. I thought maybe I can forget, but it didn't work. I was such a happy person before this. I laughed all the time, so that my husband said to me sometimes that I laughed too much. Now, however, whether I am alone or with others, in a party or a funeral, it doesn't make a difference. It's all the same to me. I live in fear. If we go out shopping, we must be back before it is dark. If my husband is not home at night, I leave the lights on. I lock all the doors, and I still can't sleep. I get distressed and become compulsive.

T: What do you do?

C: I get angry if my children don't keep quiet.

T: What do you mean by compulsion?

C: I must constantly clean and wipe and sweep. Although I've been better for about a month.

T: How long have you had this compulsions?

C: I had it since I was a child. It runs through my family.

T: You mean the compulsive cleaning?

C: Yes. For example, when we had guests and they left, I had to clean everywhere. I washed the pillowcases and the sheets. It's been a month now, though, that I don't care about cleaning anymore.

T: So you have a history of compulsive cleaning and housekeeping. What about compulsion about personal hygiene?

C: No, I don't have that. Thank God I no longer have any compulsion.

T: You said that you started locking doors when your fear started. Didn't you do it before?

C: No, not like this; it was normal. Even at nights when my husband worked at the night shift, I locked the door, said my prayers and went to bed. I woke up in the morning, listened to music, had breakfast and visited my neighbors. We talked and laughed. I was so happy and upbeat. But since my fear started, I don't care about anything. I feel high tension. It's almost as if ghosts attack me. My body starts shaking and I can't control it.

T: Tell me more about this shaking and heartbeat.

C: My body goes cold and the trembling starts from within. Or, when I remember that drug-addicted man, my heartbeat gets so fast, I feel I'm choking. My breath is stuck here (points to the upper part of her chest) and I have to take deep breaths so it gradually becomes normal again.

T: How do you sleep?

C: I took sedatives before. Although I don't take them for about a week now.

T: Do you take any other drugs?

C: I saw a psychiatrist for the fear I told you about on the phone, and he prescribed some drugs for me. I took them regularly, but I stopped the medication last week.

T: Have you visited any other specialist about your problem?

C: No, it's the first time I'm seeing a psychologist.

T: Since the fear and its consequence, the indifference, started, have you ever realized what increases them and what decreases them?

C: Nothing decreases it. It just gets worse. My family did their best. They tried taking me out, we took trips. Nothing worked.

T: They didn't have any effects?

C: No, nothing. They took me around the city and it didn't help. We went to parks and it didn't help. We took trips and it didn't help.

T: What are you afraid might happen?

C: Fear paralyzes me, my heartbeat increases and I cannot breathe.

T: What do you do then?

C: I say prayers, I recite the holy Quran. But they don't help either.

T: How is your relationship with your husband?

C: It's fine. Since my problem started, I would prefer him to go to work when it's light outside. But he leaves home at 4:20 and I am scared and cannot go back to sleep until sunrise.

T: I think your husband has arrived. I'll ask him to come in. (The husband enters with their little son. Addressing the husband) I heard the problem from your wife. I want to hear it once from you, too. (The husband describes the problem similar to what the wife said. The compulsive cleaning and the anger are also pointed out by the husband).

C: What does she do when she gets angry?

H: You can't go near her (laughing).

C: I do get angry, but it's not like I act disrespectfully, or throw things, or hit anybody. And my anger subsides immediately.

T: What makes her angry?

H: It's mainly with respect to her compulsions. If others do something that makes things dirty, and she has to clean it, she gets angry. Although her compulsions have decreased for some time now.

T: It's less, but it's still there, right?

C: For example, if we go to the park, I have to wash all the clothes when we get back. Or, if my clothes or my body touch anything in the toilet, I definitely have to take a bath and wash my clothes.

T: So the compulsions exist to some extent, right?

H: Yes.

T: What about the fear?

H: The fear has gotten worse.

T: According to what I heard, we have to treat two problems. First, the fears that have started bothering you, and then the compulsions. I want both of you to pay close attention. I am going to give you some tasks to do. You need to understand my instructions perfectly so that you can do the tasks right and get the best results.

Your first task is to stop altogether the medication you said you haven't taken for a week. Your second task is to stop doing those things which you said you did to calm yourself down, and that didn't help you. When you get better, you can recite holy Quran, and give votive offerings and do whatever you want. But now, you shouldn't do anything to try and solve your problems. Because, first, you've already done everything and seen that they don't help you; and second, the things you might do can interfere with the treatment I am going to arrange for you, so you won't get the optimum outcomes. You have done whatever you thought might help. I want you to do what I think might help you for a few weeks. Here's what you need to do: you must do a certain tasks three times a day, each time for 10 min. It's just like taking a pill three times a day. Now, what is the task? You must be alone. Nobody should interrupt you. Nothing should prevent you from doing your task. Since a month ago, certain things happened to you that scared you immensely, just as you told me. You saw certain things, you met some people under certain circumstances, and the thoughts about what you experienced enter your mind at certain times (during night time) and bother you. Within the 10-min sessions, you must remember precisely the same people, scenes and conditions, think about them and recreate them in your mind in a way as if they are actually happening. You must feel the fear and tremble with it. You must intentionally go through those conditions and experience all the trembling, paralysis, heartbeat and the choking. The more you can recreate those moods on your own, the sooner you will get well. You must make an honest effort to do the task just as I have instructed to you, so that it is precisely similar to the actual occasions when you feel the fear. You might do your best, but you fail to experience the fear just like when it takes you by surprise. You may either succeed or fail. No matter what happens, it's okay, since you have done your duty. You may even fail to recreate the mood in the first place, which is again acceptable. You may forget to do the exercise; you may oversleep; maybe you are with others and cannot do the task; it's all right. In such cases, you simply lose the task and you must not try to make up for it at some other time. You must wait for the next turn. This is because an important condition for this treatment is that you either do the exercise precisely on time, or you do not do it at all. Our next session together is in two weeks. For the first week, you must do the task three times a day, each time for 10 min. For the second week, do the task twice a day, again for 10 min. You must start from tomorrow. Now, I want you to give me three 10-min times during the day when you can sit down and do the task. I repeat: if you miss a chance, it's okay and do not try to change the time.

C: 5:00, 17:00 and 22:00 for the first week, and 5:00 and 22:00 for the second week.

T: There is one more thing you need to pay attention to. Your only task is to do the exercises according to the arrangement. You mustn't try to do anything else. You must not attempt to fight the fear at other times of the day. All I want you is to do the exercise on time and according to the instructions. The fear might come and go at other times, but you have nothing to do with them. We will talk about them later. In sum, for you to recreate the fear at those three times during the day doesn't mean that you must try to prevent them from happening at other times. Even if you want to get rid of them, you can't do it, just like you've been trying to do so unsuccessfully so far. But, it's important that you don't do anything more than what we agreed upon. See you in two weeks.

Session Two

T: It's nice to see you. Tell me what you did.

C: I lost some sessions, but I managed to do the rest. And the result was excellent. Now, I am afraid only a little bit, only a little bit. When I see drug-addicts, I act as if I haven't seen them. Thank God, I'm much better now.

T: How did you do the exercises? How did you feel within the 10 min when you were doing the exercise?

C: On the first day, my husband wasn't home and I felt sad, so I started crying. Before this, I couldn't cry no matter what I did. Then, I was able to do the exercises more easily, and it got much better.

T: Do you think you can give me a percentage of your improvement?

C: I am much better. Almost nothing is left of my problem.

T: Well, let's suppose continuing the same process can solve your problem altogether. Is there anything else you want me to help you with?

C: My compulsions with cleaning and washing.

T: Is the compulsions, which we discussed during the previous session, still with you?

H: Yes, it is.

C: It is.

T: Stick to the same exercise about recreating your fears: twice a day, each time for 5 min. When can you do them?

C: At 17:00 and 22:00.

T: Do the exercises; and we will see what happens next session.

Session Three

T: It's a pleasure to meet you again. Please tell me what you did.

C: I did the exercises more or less, by about 50%. And I feel that I am not afraid anymore and I'm cured. Now, I feel that if a drug-addicted man comes toward me, I can blow him away easily. I think it's a shame for me to be scared of drug-addicts.

T: Does that mean the fear has kept decreasing, as you reported the previous session, and hasn't increased in any way?

C: Yes, it has decreased, and I feel no fear anymore.

T: Well, we are done with the fears and you don't have a problem anymore. Now, we need a schedule for dealing with the compulsions. Since our summer holidays start tomorrow, and we can't have sessions together, we postpone the schedule to the autumn. We have 3 months until then. Within this time, we can see how the treatment of your fears turn out, and we can get ready for the treatment of your compulsions. You no longer need to do any exercises, and the fears are not supposed to bother you anymore. But, if it so happens that after, say, a month you experience the fears again, first give them some time. If they do not go away after a couple of days, you can make a schedule similar to what we had together on your own. You agree to do the task at three times every day from the next day. You must arrange three fixed times for doing the tasks, just like what we did here. You recreate your fears. If you do the exercises according to my instructions, you will get the same results within a week.

17.3 Assessment of Treatment Outcome and Follow-Up

The course of the treatment was completed in 3 sessions. Assessment of the treatment outcome, which was based on the patients' comments in a graded scale of 0–100 and an open-ended question, indicated 100% recovery. A 3-year follow-up evaluation showed no relapse.

18 Client #16 (Female, 12 Years Old, Single)

18.1 Case Introduction

NA a 12 years old girl came to the University of Tehran Clinic with her elder brother because of her paralyses symptoms following through medical examinations which excluded a physical cause of her symptoms. She developed the paralysis of her feet, mostly in her left foot, at age of 8 first. Then the symptoms progressed to her left hand and got worsened gradually. NA is the last child of a family of 6 living in a village. NA is described as dependent to her mother. Her mother also has had the same problem since the age of 13; a kind of conversion disorder that she adapted to. The clinical interview based on DSM-5 (APA 2013), showed that NA had the criteria for conversion disorder. This is her first visit for psychological treatment. NA was seen for 7 sessions over a period of 15 weeks.

18.2 Course of Treatment

Session One

Therapist (T): (After the greetings and the social stage of the interview) please tell me why you are here.

Client (C): When I walk, my toes fold inwards, which make my legs ache. If I sit down for several minutes and don't walk, they become normal again. This problem goes to other parts of my body. It suddenly goes to my head, and then moves to my shoulders. Then it goes into my hands and my hands become locked and I can't move them (points to his left hand). Suddenly, my left leg feels sore and I can't walk. When I'm standing up, I can't control myself, and I move. I can't stand up straight.

T: What do you mean you move?

Senior Brother (SB): She cannot concentrate. She moves her legs and sways from side to side.

C: I've visited many specialists in the past three to four years. I did tests too. Some say it's kidney infection, and some say I have some kind of blood problem.

SB: I have to add that our mother's legs have the exact same problem. She believes that there is this wind (a term in traditional medicine) in her body that enters her hand sometimes and makes it numb. Sometimes, it goes to her waits and legs. My sister's problem is that the tip of her toes are directed inward as she walks (just like my mother), and she cannot walk after taking some steps (pointing to her feet that come together at the toes and create an angle). It then gets impossible for her to walk. If she tries too hard to put her toes straight, it gets really painful. We visited many specialists and she has had several tests. Drug therapy had the opposite result and made it worse.

T: What did they say the problem was?

SB: The orthopedic tests showed that there was nothing wrong with her legs. They said that she needed more calcium and vitamins, and she took them. But it didn't work. Her problem was

M. A. Besharat, *Paradoxical Psychotherapy: A Practitioner's Guide*,
University of Tehran Science and Humanities Series,
https://doi.org/10.1007/978-3-031-27717-7_18

less serious three years ago, but it got worse and worse gradually. She is highly dependent on my mother. This was why I convinced her to go to a boarding school (there are schools in several provinces that accept top students from nearby villages so as to offer them a better educational atmosphere) so that she can be away from mother and learn to be more independent.

T: (Addressing the client) Is your brother right?

C: Yes.

T: Do you all live together?

C: Yes.

T: How many brothers and sisters do you have?

C: There are four of us; one brother and three sisters.

T: This is your brother, and are you the last child?

C: Yes.

T: You said that your problem started three to four years ago. Did you notice, then, that your mother had a similar problem?

C: Yes. When mother wakes up in the morning, she is fine. But after working for some time, she becomes tired and she needs to get some rest, like me, so as to be fine again.

T: Are you like that, too?

C: Yes.

T: So, you are fine from morning to noon, and…?

C: When I've had some sleep and rest, I'm fine and I can walk easily.

T: What happens after that?

C: Then my hands become all stiff, and I can't move them.

T: Does your hand become stiff suddenly?

C: Yes.

T: Is it the left hand mainly?

C: Yes, it's also the right hand, but mainly the left.

T: You said that first your foot becomes stiff (C: Yes.), and then your hand (C: Yes). Does this always happen in the same order? (C: Yes.) So it's first your fott, then your hand and then your head, right?

C: Yes, these parts of my head (points to some spots on her forehead).

T: How long is your headache?

C: 10 min.

T: What about your hand (pointing to her left hand)?

C: At first, it was just my left foot, and my hand was fine. Then, I visited a doctor who prescribed drugs for me, and then my left hand got stiff too.

T: You said that when you were coming here, it was difficult for you to walk here from about 100 m away. What about before that?

SB: We came here with a taxi, and then we walked here from about 100 m away. At first, she tried to put her feet straight, but she couldn't. At the end of the way, it was really difficult for her, because her feet had become bent.

T: (Addressing the client) Do you feel it yourself?

C: Yes, I want to put my feet straight, but my feet hurt and I can't do it.

T: You have done tests and it has turned out that there is no blood or orthopedic problems. Does anyone else other than you and your mother suffer from a similar problem in your family?

SB: No, it's just her and our mother.

T: Dependency on the mother! How could you bear to get away from your mother and go to the boarding school?

C: The first couple of days were difficult. But there were other girls there. We became friends, and it was all right after that.

SB: She also had a close friend. They were together from the first to the fifth grade, and they were accepted in the boarding school together. I think one of the reasons she wanted to go to the boarding school was that she didn't want to leave her friend.

T: What happens if I say that you shouldn't go to the boarding school anymore?

C: (Surprised) You mean I shouldn't study anymore?

T: No, you still study, but not at a boarding school. Isn't there a school in your own village?

SB: There is one in a nearby village.

C: I can do it, if I there are relatives in that village I can go to.

SB: Our grandparents live in that village, and we had enrolled her in that school at first. But then, we took her to that boarding school.

T: I believe you had better not study at a boarding school, so that you can visit your mother once or twice a week, whenever you like. I believe that you should definitely study school, but you can go to a school close to your own village and study there. This way, you can spend more time with your mother. If this is part of my treatment for you to get well, can you accept it and do it?

C: (Passionately[1]) Yes, yes.

T: Yes?

C: Yes.

T: (There are discussion about other matters such as how she can change her school and come back home.) Has the problem with your hands and feet become less or more severe within the last four years? I want to know whether you can tell me what conditions make it worse or better.

C: Yes, there are times when I walk a lot and I have no difficulty. However, at other times I feel the pain although I haven't walked that much.

T: Have you ever tried to understand why you feel the pain sometimes, although you haven't walked that much, and you don't feel it at other times despite the fact that you have walked a lot? (This question is put forward in a number of different ways. Finally, it is concluded that when the client is under stress, the problem becomes more noticeable. On the other hand, at time when she is happy and calm, the problem goes away). As the client puts it herself, "whenever I'm upset, my hands and feet are upset as well. And when I'm happy, my body is happy and at rest."

T: Who can give you this happiness more than anyone else?

C: My mother.

T: How does she do that?

C: (Passionately) I love my mother so much. When I am with my mother, I am happy.

T: What about when you are away from your mother?

C: I keep telling myself I have to separate from my mother sooner or later. I try to soothe myself and help myself tolerate being away from her. I can be with my mother this year, and the next year. But what if I enter the university and have to leave, like my brother? So I have to be strong (she mentions several rational reasons that are mainly influenced by the advice given to her by her brother, and is situated at the exact opposite of her genuine emotions and affects).

T: This is a good idea, and this is why your brother suggested that you go to a boarding school so that you can become more independent. However, it is too early for you. You must follow my orders so that the problem is solved. Then, we can think about becoming more independent.

Who makes you feel calm, other than your mother?

C: (Pointing to her brother) My brother.

T: What about your father?

C: He is also good.

T: And the rest of your family?

C: They are also fine. When we are together, and we talk and laugh and are happy, my hands and feet are happy too and aren't painful.

T: Do you take any drugs?

C: No.

T: Remember that as long as you are coming to me, you don't need to take any drugs nor should you visit any other specialist. When you go back home, leave the boarding school and go to the school near home. Then, do your best to go back home at nights, unless you can't make it. It's up to you. (addressing the brother) You shouldn't tell her what to do. (addressing the client) You should decide when to go back home, and when to stay at your grandparents'. The only

[1] According to clinical findings and based on theories of normal developmental processes, early separation from the mother can be traumatic, especially for children who are dependent on their mothers to some extent. Such a separation, at its best, sacrifices the individual's emotional capital for achieving educational success. Such a success is still possible without the separation as long as the individual has the capacity and aptitude for it. Psychological disorder is one of the consequences of such a sacrificing. For this reason, and due to systemic reasons of the treatment, this reunion is part of the process of the PTC model. It is a structural technique that can both prevent possible psychological traumas in the future, and is necessary for treating the patient's hysterical paralysis at present.

one making a decision about it is you not your grandparents, your parents or your brother. Only you![2] On what days do you have to go to school?

C: Saturday to Wednesday.

T: And what hours?

C: It starts at 7:30 to 13:30.

T: When do you wake up in the morning?

C: I wake up at 4 in the morning in order to study.

T: Do you sleep well at nights?

C: Yes.

T: Do you eat well?

C: Yes.

T: That's great. You wake up early and you have enough time to study and do other things. This helps you to be able to do what I suggest you to, so your problem can be solved. Let's suppose that you can move from the boarding school to the school close to your home in a week. After that, I want you to do the followings: every day, you should act as if you have the pain in your hands and feet for about 15 to 20 min (the time for doing the exercise is thirty minutes after waking up). You are like an actress on the stage of the theater. You have 15 to 20 min to play the role of yourself, when you are walking and your feet bend inwards. You take a few steps, it becomes difficult for you to walk, you feel the pain in your feet, your hands become stiff and you can't move them. You must play all the pain and stiffness you've been experiencing for four years within the 15 to 20 min. You must act as if you really feel the pain and the stiffness in your hands and feet and you cannot move them. If you can play as if you are really feeling it, you will get the best outcome. We will have our next session in three weeks. The first week is for you to change your school. You start the exercise from the second week. During the first week, do the exercise every day except for Friday, and during the second week, do it every day except for Thursday and Friday. Pay attention that I only ask you to do the exercise at the time we have agreed. This does not mean that you should try to fight the pain and the stiffness at other times. You don't think about other times. Live your normal life, and let the pain and the stiffness come and go. We will talk about it the next session.

Session Two

T: Welcome. Please tell me what you did. You were supposed to change schools first, and then there were a series of exercises I had asked you to do. Did you change your school?

SB: Yes, we did.

T: Are you satisfied with this change?

C: Yes, it's fine.

T: When did you move to the new school?

C: Three weeks ago, after we left here.

T: How did you do with the exercises?

C: I did them in the mornings, as you ordered.

T: So, tell me what happened when you did the exercise, went to school and then spent the rest of your day?

C: I went to school and came back home. I rested a little, and then I studied my lessons.

T: Where did you stay at nights?

C: I stayed at my grandparents', and went back home on Thursdays and Fridays. There was a holiday in the middle of the week, and I went back home again.

T: How were your hand and feet during the day?

C: The pains and stiffness's have become much less.

T: Can you compare them to when you still hadn't come here?

C: They were less than before.

T: Can you give me a percentage?

C: 60% less.

T: Do you mean that you still feel the pain and the stiffness by 40%?

C: I only felt them once during the last three weeks.

T: You didn't feel them at all on the other days?

C: I did, but it was very little. Just once, it was a little severe.

[2] This emphasis on the client being the sole decision-maker in this regard, can prepare the ground for subsequent psychotherapeutic changes that come after the treatment of hysterical paralysis and are targeted at the client's sense of dependency/ independency. These are interventions carried out within the framework of the PTC model, with the intention of treating personality problems and disorders.

T: So, we can say that the problem was not noticeable during the three weeks, except for that one single day, when it caused you pain. Is that right?

C: Yes.

T: (Addressing the brother) What do you think?

C: I wasn't with her all this time. But we walked a distance together, and I felt that she could walk better than before.

T: Okay. I'd said that you mustn't do the exercise during the Friday of the second week, and the Thursday and Friday of the third week. Did you do it?

C: Yes, I did not do the exercise on those days.

T: How did you feel on the days you didn't do the exercise?

C: I was fine, like the rest of the days.

T: Do you study well?

C: Yes. I wake up early in the morning and start studying.

T: Congratulations, both because you study hard, and because you have made progress with respect to your problem. Improvement by 60% during the first stage of the treatment is excellent. Actually, I think it is more than 60% if you felt the pain only on one day. Compared to before when you felt it every day, it can be said that the percentage is greater than 60. Anyway, the main part of the problem is solved, and now you know the way to solve your problem. Now, we only need to exercise a little bit more, so that the process of treatment is complete. Before we move on, tell me more about your hands and head.

C: My hand was totally fine, and my head was painful only over here (points to a spot on her forehead).

T: Your hand has been fine, and the pain in your head is limited to that spot; when you study your lessons. What kind of a pain is it? Is it just that part, or all your head?

C: Yes, it's just this part.

T: When does this pain start?

C: Around noon, and afterwards.

T: When does it increase?

C: When there's a lot of noise.

T: Any kind of noise, whether it is at school or elsewhere?

C: Yes, any kind, anywhere.

T: When is it at its worst?

C: At school.

T: How long does it take?

C: Sometimes until night, and sometimes till the next morning.

T: If you feel the pain till the next morning, does it affect your school?

C: When it's with me until the next morning, it goes away when I wake up. And I don't feel it during school.

T: Do you feel it every day, or sometimes?

C: Sometimes.

T: Compared to the past, has this headache increased, decreased or remained the same?

C: It has become less than before.

T: You still should decide on your own whether to go back home, or stay at your grandparents'. You don't need to do the exercise on Thursdays and Fridays. During the week, do the exercise on even days (Saturday, Monday and Wednesday). Don't let the exercise exceed 15 min each time. It's okay if it's less than 15 min, but it mustn't be more than that. You don't need to do anything special about your headache, at present.

Session Three

T: It's nice to see you again. It's been a month since our last session. Please tell me what you did with the exercises.

C: I did them.

T: How were your hands, feet and head?

C: They were good, but not as good as the first three weeks. There was less improvement.

T: So, you had improvement similar to the previous session when you said you had 60% improvement. Only it was less than that time. Is that right?

C: It was 40% this time.

T: So there was improvement, only slower. Last session, you said that the problem was painful for only one day, and you were fine for the rest of the days.

C: This time I felt severe pain only for a day.

T: Which day was it?

C: It was Sunday.

T: What time was it?

C: It was about 7:30 when I wanted to go to school.

T: What was the day three weeks ago when you felt the pain?

C: That was Wednesday.

T: Why do you think it was Sunday, and not some other day? Can you guess?

C: I think because Sunday is an odd day, when I don't have to do the exercise. That's why it got worse.

T: You said that it was severe for one day. What about all the other days?

C: It was medium during the rest of the days.

T: What about the rest of the days of the first three weeks?

C: It was low during those days, but it was medium during the last four weeks.

T: So, this was about your feet. What about your hand (pointing to the left hand)?

C: My hand doesn't have a problem anymore.

T: Can we say that you no longer suffered from the problem in your hand from the very beginning?

C: Yes, my hand has been fine ever since.

T: And your head?

C: I felt the headache at school, sometimes.

T: How is it at school, with your lessons, and your friends?

C: It is good.

SB: She is a top student. The only reason the school agrees to us coming to these sessions is that she studies hard and her teacher and the whole school like her.

T: You didn't take any drugs during this time, right? Because we agreed that you mustn't take drugs.

C: No, I didn't.

T: Do 10-min exercises for the first five days of the next two weeks, before you go to school in the morning. The exercise can be no more than 10 min. After two weeks, you will give me a report on what you have done through the phone, and then we will decided what you should do next. Since you live far-away, and you are a student, we do part of our job through the phone.

Session Four

T: Welcome. A long time has passed since our last two sessions and the phone call. Tell me what you did.

C: I was fine during the first three weeks. Then, for four weeks, my feet went stiff for half of the day. And I felt better during the last weeks.

T: In general, through the last three weeks, to what extent were your feet stiff, and fine? Tell me in percentage terms.

C: During these nine weeks, they were fine by 40%, and stiff by 60%.

T: What about your hand?

C: My hand has been fine ever since.

T: And your head?

C: I headache during the first week after I left here. Then, there was no headache anymore.

T: You said that in some cases, your foot was stiff by 60%. Was there a difference between Thursdays and Fridays and other days of the week?

C: It was better on Thursdays and Fridays.

T: What do you think was difference between days of the week that made your foot more or less painful and stiff?

C: I think it can because of the pressure of school.

T: The interval between last session and this session became so long because of your exams. Are there any more exams left?

C: There is, one more.

T: (Addressing the brother) Do you want to add anything?

SB: I was here in the city most of the time and wasn't with her. But, in general, my family thinks she has made good progress.

T: During what part of the day were your foot stiff mostly?

C: It was mainly noon till night.

T: Thanks for your report. You have made good improvement so far. At the same time, the stress caused by school exams were influential upon your condition. Also, you have no longer had pain in your hand and head. We need to make a change to our timetable, till the next session. Do the exercise for five minutes on even days, before going to school. And on odd days, which are Sundays and Tuesdays, do it at noon (according to her school schedule, it was agreed that she can do the exercise at 12 when she goes home to have lunch. Students have to go back to school after lunch, and have classes till 15). Also, focus the exercises on your feet. You no longer need the exercise for the hand. Call me in two weeks, so that we can see what to do next.

Session Five

T: It's nice to see you. Again, a long time has passed since our last session together. Tell me what happened during this interval.

C: I did the exercises. But I've become worse since last session.

T: What do you mean by worse?

C: I was fine at morning when I went to school. But my feet went stiff in the afternoon when I came back home.

T: It can therefore be said that you have become worse compared to the earlier sessions, but you are still better than before you came here.

C: Yes, I'm still better than before. But compared to the earlier sessions, when my feet did not have much pain, I am worse.

T: Why do you think it is that you haven't become better sine three months ago?

C: I think it's because the lessons are too difficult. Any time there was a difficult exam, I felt more pain and stiffness in my feet. Sometime, when I walk a lot, it gets worse.

T: How long is it okay for you to walk before your feet start to ache?

C: I can walk up to 20 min, and there will be no problem. But if I walk more than that, they'll get sore.

T: Since March, have there been times when you didn't have the problem? For example the days when you were with your mother, or you were happy?

C: No, I've had it every day.

T: What does your family think? What would they have said about your condition, if they were here right now?

C: They think that I don't do your exercises, and that's why I'm not better.

T: But you do the exercises, right?

C: Yes.

T: Who keeps reminding you to do the exercises more than others?

C: My mother says "do the doctor's orders so you get better."

T: What does your brother say?

C: He says "do it as you like."

T: Your condition isn't good right now. What do you think will happen if it gets worse?

C: I won't be able to walk anymore.

T: Has it ever happened to you? Have you ever been unable to walk?

C: There are time when I have to stop during my walk, but I still could do it.

T: What do others do at school, when you feel bad and can't walk easily?

C: They tell me to stop for a minute and rest, and then keep on walking.

T: How are the teachers? Do they know about your problem?

C: No, they don't.

T: Where were during the New Year holidays and what did you do?

C: I was fine for one day, but I didn't feel well for the rest of the days.

T: How is your hand?

C: My hand is not stiff anymore.

T: And your head?

C: I have headache at times when there is too much noise.

T: What else do you think can help your feet to get better?

C: Rest and taking a bath help a little. I don't think there is anything else that can help.

T: (The brother enters the session and is addressed) Tell me what you think about her condition since March?

SB: I was mostly here in the city, at work. I went back home during the New Year holidays. I have realized that when my sister is being watched by someone, her feet become stiff, but she is fine when no one is watching her. She is completely normal. Both I and my father have seen this. And when she makes a conscious effort to put her feet down correctly, it gets even worse. If she is in a situation when she pays no attention to her walking, she can walk normally, without any problems. Also, her walking style and her condition completely match those of my mother.

T: You just heard what your brother said. Do you agree with him?

C: Yes, he is right.

T: (Addressing the brother) How did your sister walk during the holidays when you were home?

SB: It was only on the thirteenth when she was wearing special type of shoes so as to climb the mountain, that she had difficulty walking. I didn't see a problem on other days and she was able to walk normally, more or less. It was only the thirteenth, and I think it was because of the shoes, rather than her feet.

T: Do you agree with your brother that there was no problem, generally, during the holidays?

C: Yes.

T: So when was the time it got worse?

C: That was only when I walked a lot.

(Taking into account the client's personal tendency for educational success, the establishment of perfectionist standards and expectations by the family, especially by the mother, the client and the family were given the necessary training for removing pointless pressure and stress. It was also decided that the client must get one more hour of rest during the day. Visits to the family increased from once every two weeks to once a week. She was asked to do the exercises after taking the bath (the client takes a bath three times a week), as long as 5 to 10 min.

Session Six

T: (The client's mother and brother are present during the session.) Welcome! (addressing the mother) thank you for accepting to come here. I would like to know what you think about your daughter's condition.

Mother (M): "L" was fine until the third grade. When she was in the fourth grade, one day I saw she was putting her feet down on the ground in an angled way. "Walk properly. Why are you walking like that?" I asked her. Then, her father saw it too, and we took her to a doctor. She hasn't been cured ever since (the rest of the report given by the mother resembles the reports given by the brother and the client).

T: Now let's hear "L" tells us about her present condition. Tell me what you did during the last two weeks.

C: I did all the exercises you prescribed for me to do, but it didn't work and my feet still have the same problem.

SB: My sister no longer suffers from the hand, the neck and the head problems. But I think the pain in her foot (left foot) has gotten worse. We were coming here today. I looked at her feet and realized that she put her feet down in a zigzag manner. Her feet landed in front of one another, and it was really difficult to walk that way.

T: How have others reacted to her condition? I mean the other family members.

SB: My mother is really impatient about her problem and expects her to get well immediately. She even argues with her about it. She thinks that she does it on purpose! One of our sisters thinks, however, that "L" is not doing it on purpose. She cannot walk normally. She would if she could.

T: (Addressing the brother) What do you think?

SB: I don't think she is doing it on purpose, either. I think we must wait for "L" to complete her treatment so that she can get well completely. We shouldn't expect her to get well immediately. But my mother prefers her to suddenly get well, even if by taking some medication.

T: (Addressing the client) And what do you think?

C: I think that it's not up to me. I do my best and I like to get well, but I can't.

T: (Addressing the mother) I've heard you have a similar problem in your back. Is that right?

M: I didn't have any problem till I was 13. We wove carpets in those days. I woke up one morning and I realized that I couldn't control my legs. I couldn't move my arms and legs. We went to a doctor and … (The mother has always had to work hard for long hours, due to living in the village. She is 45 now and she has adapted herself to the problem more or less, and she has no inner motivation to treat her problem. Her usual way of dealing with the problem is that she takes a rest every once in a while so that the pain and the stiffness would go away. She believes, in line with traditional medicine, that there is some wind in her back that causes this problem).

T: (Addressing the mother) L's problem is not of the sort to be solved through medication. You know that she had given several tests and has taken lots of drugs.

M: She has had 25 different types of tests, and has taken a lot of medication. But she hasn't gotten any better.

T: The nature of her condition is so that it cannot be cured through medication, as you have experience yourself. Her problem must be solved in another way. We need your cooperation in order to be able to solve it. The only reason I asked you to come here, despite all the difficulties of traveling long distances, was that I wanted you to hear it from me yourself and help us. You are not responsible for treating L. She is an intelligent girl and understands everything. She is concerned more than you or anyone else about her health, future, and happiness. You are a mother and you feel responsible about your daughter's future. That's great. However, in order to help L become better, we must all help one another. And the only help we can give is to hold L herself responsible for her feet. Her brother is simply being kind enough to bring her here and take her back home. He doesn't interfere in the process of her treatment in any other way. None of the family members, and more specifically you—the mother-, must not meddle in the treatment of L's condition. Any interference, comment or question on your part can make the process of treatment longer and more difficult. Her brother brings her here, I monitor her progress and she is the one responsible for her treatment. No one else should say anything. The main reason I invited you here was to ask you this. I wanted you to hear it directly from me, and I hope you do as I have asked you to.

(Addressing the client) Your task is to go back home every weekend, and when you are there, you must do your best to have the problem in your feet. In other words, if your feet are stiff for four hours a day, you better try to make it five, six or seven hours, or even the entire day. Make no attempt to put your feet straight on the ground. Even if you can walk straight, try to bend your feet inwards and walk that way. Your mother is here and hears our talk. I have asked her to have nothing to do with your feet. Even if she sees you walk normally, she can say "didn't the doctor ask you to walk that way?" She cannot tell you, however, to put your feet down in a zigzag manner. (addressing the mother) Can you follow my order?

M: Yes.

T: (Addressing the mother) I thank you for attending this session. All I wanted was for you to come here and hear the order directly from me, so that you follow it. From now on, no one from L's family has anything to do with the problem of her feet. L is the one responsible for the treatment of her feet and she will do so under my supervision. We have agreed that she must go back home during the weekend and try her best to walk in the worst manner possible. I also ask you to not go to L during the week, and simply wait for her to come home at the end of the week (according to the report given by the client, the mother goes to visit her sometimes). As for her lessons, I have told her what to do so as not to feel any stress about school. Stress can make the problem of her feet get worse, so you must not talk to her about her lessons either. L is a great student who studies hard without anyone telling her what to do. During the schooldays, do the exercises about your feet and your walking 5 min before getting ready to go to school.

Session Seven

T: Welcome back! A long time has passed since we had our last session. Where are you now, and what do you do?

C: I'm in the 8th grade in my village.

T: How is school?

C: It's fine, and I do well.

T: That's good. How about your feet?

C: I still have that old problem with my feet. My hands and my head, however, have been treated ever since.

T: (Addressing the brother) You told me over the phone that a new series of tests were done on L, and the doctors have confirmed that she doesn't suffer from a physical problem, and the cause of her condition is psychological. (addressing L) What do you have to say about it?

C: We visited some other doctors, and had some tests. They had different comments. One of them said that my problem is definitely a hereditary one which doesn't have a cure. I can only prevent it from getting worse through taking medication, drinking milk and wearing special shoes. I tried all of them. There was also an injection which didn't help at all. But there was a capsule which, when I had it and then drank some milk on the same day, I felt better. Special shoes have also helped me a little.

T: All right. You checked and realized that when you take the capsule and drink some milk, it helps you. But it didn't help when you didn't drink milk afterwards?

C: That's right.

T: Did you keep taking the capsule and the milk for, like, a month or two to see whether it helped your feet?

C: No, I didn't do that.

T: Well, let me ask you this my good girl: if the capsule and milk helped you, why didn't you take them for a longer time?

SB: The problem of her feet still emerged after 3 in the afternoon, even though she took the capsule and milk.

C: I couldn't stop that.

T: After what you just told me, I am more certain than ever that your problem is not a medical one (though I would like your brother to ask the name of the medical condition from that specialist and tell it to me). You have so far visited many specialists. Except for one of them, all the rest confirmed that your problem is a psychological one. And that one specialist has told you that your problem is hereditary, and cannot be cured. You have kept asking him to give you a prescription, and he has prescribed something for you. But I think even you yourself know that it is not going to work. Otherwise, you would have kept taking the capsule. So, don't bother yourself any further. Enough with the medical tests and cures. As long as you think about medical solutions, you can't be helped through psychological treatment. I did my best to put an end to others' interventions, especially your mother's. I don't know how successful I've been and to what extent you have followed my orders. I tried, from the first day, to make you understand that you are the only who must assume the responsibility of your treatment. I told you that you must decide on yourself whether to go back to your mother or not. I wanted you to learn to assume responsibility for your personal life. We did all that so you stop expecting help from others, be it medical doctors, other specialists or family members. Even I myself tried to move to the background, telling you I'm only here to supervise your progress. Why did I do this? Because this problem is of a nature, a psychological nature, that cannot be solved as long you don't rely on yourself and yourself alone. As long as you invest hope in others and expect them to find you a solution, as long as you look for some drug to help you get better, there will be no change. As you can see, there hasn't been any change. You can only invest hope in your own efforts, which must be made under my supervision. Fortunately, time has worked to your advantage. Now that you have grown older, you both understand what I tell you better, and be more prepared to assume responsibility.

In case you agree to not take any other interventions, and give up hope in a medical solution, we can begin our work again. You can do the exercises twice a day: one at 6:30 before getting ready to go to school, and the other one at 17:00 when you are back from school and has had a rest. In both times, spend no more than 10 min to do the exercises about the stiffness of your feet, bending your feet inwards and walking in a zigzag manner. Recreate and re-experience any other problems you feel with respect to your feet during the exercises. Do the exercises every day for two weeks. During the third week up to our next session, do them only on even days (Saturday, Monday and Wednesday). You don't need to do the exercise when you go home to your parents.

18.3 Assessment of Treatment Outcome and Follow-Up

The course of the treatment was not completed. Assessment of the treatment outcome for the first 7 sessions, which was based on the patients' comments in a graded scale of 0–100 and an open-ended question, indicated 50% recovery. A 19-month follow-up evaluation indicated that there was no relapse concerning the 50% improvement. However, the other 50% requires the treatment to be completed.[3]

[3] Taking into account the evidence gathered from the reports given by the client, and the treatment outcomes achieved in general (with respect to the hands, the feet and the head), and the completed treatment of hysterical paralyses in the hand and the head, the cause of the client's hysterical paralysis in the feet was diagnosed to be her dependence on her mother as well as her dependent personality characteristics in general. On the other hand, continuing systemic intervention was not possible due to the distance and the incomplete cooperation on the part of the mother, who was the most important member of the system and the target of the client's dependency (pay attention to the heightened role of the value of the disease, especially based on the report given in session six). For the above reasons, the main treatment method to be adopted with respect to the client is modifying her personality characteristics.

Client #17 (Male, 23 Years Old, Single) 19

19.1 Case Introduction

Mr. HA, a 23-year-old student, was referred to the University of Tehran Clinic because of his clinical depression. He developed his psychological problems 5 years ago starting with anxiety first. HA visited a psychiatrist for his anxiety disorder, and took anti-anxiety medications with a good outcome removing his anxiety. Three years later he developed his depression which continued till now: "I feel empty, I have no goal to follow and I have lost all my motivation. What upsets me the most is that I was a capable person who made good decisions and set ambitious goals". Then he received anti-depressant medications without any improvement. The clinical interview based on DSM-5 (APA 2013), showed that HA had the criteria for major depressive disorder. HA's clinical condition had a great impact on his study as well as his relationships with the opposite sex. This is his first visit to receive psychological treatment. HA was seen for 6 sessions over a period of 14 weeks.

19.2 Course of Treatment

Session One

Therapist (T): (After greetings and the social stage of the interview) Please tell me why you are here.

Client (C): I started suffering from anxiety since the year I had the university entrance exam. I went to a psychiatrist who prescribed anti-anxiety medications for me. I took the medication and the anxiety went away. I was accepted in the entrance exam and entered university. I had a hard time in the dormitory, but I pulled myself up to term 5. However, I had lost all motivation by the time I reached the fifth term. I left my studies and I failed the term. I continued over the same line up to term 7, when the pressure and the stress of failing the term (if I failed one more term, I would have been expelled) brought back the anxiety I had endured several years before. I went to the psychiatrist again and went through drug therapy, but I didn't get a result. This time, there were lack of motivation and purposelessness added to my anxiety. I failed term 7, unfortunately, and only could escape being expelled through providing medical documents for my problems. I am still a student, but these problems really disturb me. I feel empty, I have no goal to follow and I have lost all my motivation. What upsets me the most is that I was a capable person who made good decisions and set ambitious goals. Right now, however, try to think of my old goals to follow again, it's almost as if someone comes out of me after a week and removes all those goals from my mind and then I lost all motivation and purpose again. The state of losing motivation and purpose continues for about four months till I can again be able to pull

M. A. Besharat, *Paradoxical Psychotherapy: A Practitioner's Guide*,
University of Tehran Science and Humanities Series,
https://doi.org/10.1007/978-3-031-27717-7_19

myself together, wake up and form a set of goals from scratch. But after a week, everything goes blank in my mind and I lost purpose and motivation. It's almost I forget everything and must start from scratch. I have done this so often that I think I no longer have control over anything and this duality really bothers me. My third problem is desire for the opposite sex, both sexually and emotionally, which I think has been a negative influence.

T: What do you mean by an influence?

C: It has preoccupied my mind for the most part. I never could form successful relationships with the opposite sex, which drove me toward masturbation.

T: By negative influence, you mean that the opposite sex has occupied all your mind and thought, is that right?

C: Yes, totally occupied.

T: And you haven't been able to form a real relationship?

C: Yes, I think because I have had no experience in this regard before entering university, I do not have the skills and the ability to form relationships.

T: Well, we will get back to it later. You mentioned some inner duality before. What did you mean? Do you feel that your mind goes blank, or do you feel there is someone who wipes your mind clean?

C: I feel there is someone else living inside my mind, apart from me, and the reason I have given up on everything is that I feel this second person is much stronger than me and I have no chance against him. When I create some framework within my mind to follow, he comes along and destroys the framework completely, making me feel lost and helpless. I escape myself for two to three months before the circumstances can make me ready for creating another framework.

T: Do you think there is someone else who comes along and removes the things you have created in your mind?

C: Exactly.

T: What do you mean by someone else? You need to help me understand the problem. Who is this person? How does he enter your mind?

C: Maybe he is the lazy part of me who comes along and takes control over the active part.

T: You mean that person is another aspect of you?

C: Yes, another stronger aspect of me, who takes control of me.

T: Do you think we better call him another aspect of yourself, or a whole other person with an independent existence?

C: No, I'm sure he is another aspect of me.

T: Let me recapitulate this dual aspect, see if I have gotten it right. You are of the opinion that you are two people; one who creates, and another one who destroys.

C: This is a more precise way of putting it.

T: You mean you are two people, someone who builds and another one who annihilates?

C: It's exactly so. And when he destroys things, my mind becomes totally blank before I gradually build it again.

T: Do you need some time to be able to build it again?

C: Yes, and that's what really bothers me.

T: We can say that this time is filled with lack of motivation and purposelessness, right?

C: Exactly. I feel a total lack of motivation in this interval.

T: Between these two persons, who is the stronger of the two?

C: I think the one who destroys.

T: It seems so. The destroyer is stronger than the builder.

C: That's right.

T: And we need to reinforce the builder.

C: I tried so much to do so, but I haven't been successful.

T: What did you do?

C: I think about it a lot. I write down everything I have created in my mind, so that I have them before my eyes and follow them. I even begin following them, but then he comes along and destroys everything, and I retreat like a loser. I no longer see what I have written down before my eyes, and I don't follow them, which is the lack of motivation.

T: You talked about some anxiety that started before the university exam and then came back to you during the university years. What were its characteristics?

C: The year I had the university entrance exam, I suddenly felt anxiety. I was restless and couldn't calm down. I couldn't focus for studying, and I left home.

T: Do you know why this anxiety overcame you all of a sudden?

C: No. Everything was fine up to that point.

T: How old were you then?

C: Eighteen.

T: What else was there apart from the restlessness? Fear, worry,...?

C: There was extreme fear; fear of failing the exam, fear of the future, of my family and my relatives.

T: Did you ever have a similar experience before you had the anxiety for the university exam?

C: No anxiety at all. Everything was so normal.

T: So, it was your first time. As for the symptoms of that anxiety, you mentioned restlessness. You went to a doctor, took some medication and got better. And you mentioned that the anxiety came back in university. Tell me about it.

C: I was fine at the beginning of entering university. I took a lot of courses. My friends warned me against it, but I was so confident that I did it anyway. I believed that I was able to pass them with great marks. The anxiety started from later September. This time it was so intense, and I also felt extreme restlessness and lack of concentration. I didn't want to take drugs this time. I tried so hard not to take drugs, but I gave in and went to a psychiatrist.

T: What were the symptoms this time?

C: Extreme restlessness and a series of negative feelings. My neck goes stiff and I feel as if blood doesn't run through my veins. When it gets worse, my heart beat increases insanely. My mind is full of negative thoughts in such circumstances. I am in the lowest depths of hopelessness, emptiness and lack of motivation. These come to my mind involuntarily.

T: You said that you took drugs the last time you felt the anxiety in university. However, the lack of motivation is with you still.

C: Extreme lack of motivation, emptiness and purposelessness.

T: Can you eat and sleep well in such times?

C: I can't sleep well at all. I am awake until 4:00 to 5:00 in the morning. It was almost as if I was afraid of sleep and escaped it.

T: Did you actually escape it, or did you want to go to sleep but couldn't?

C: No, I escaped it.

T: Why?

C: Because if I went to sleep, I would wake up in a bad mood and would have to take drugs.

T: What woke you up?

C: The stiffness in the neck.

T: Did you escape sleep so you can remain awake and have your medication on time, or what?

C: To avoid having it happen to me in sleep. Because when it happened during sleep, I woke up with the most intense negative feelings.

T: Didn't it happen when you were awake?

C: When I was awake I could immediately take drugs if I felt that anxiety was coming.

T: Did you mean lack of motivation and purposelessness when you mentioned negative feelings at sleep?

C: Yes, and they were with me the whole day and preoccupied my mind.

T: How have you been during the past month?

C: Failing the term was a huge pressure on me. As time went by, and they accepted my medical documents, I felt better and I have decreased my drugs from 7 to 4 a day. But I feel I can't pull myself together and take care of my life. Maybe I am worried that if I want to start doing things seriously, the anxiety may come back. Maybe the laziness and lack of motivation are only here to keep me away from the anxiety. I am afraid it may come back and overwhelm me.

T: Do you have to go to classes right now, in university?

C: Yes.

T: Let's review what we have discussed so far, so we can start our job. I believe that we better not talk about the third problem and steer clear of relationships and sexuality. We can get to them later on when we have dealt with other problems.

C: Yes, I agree. Because that's not my main problem right now.

T: You need to do an exercise up until our next session, which will be in two weeks. The exercise consists of playing a role for 10 min, according to my instruction. You find a place where you can be alone and concentrate without anything to interrupt you. The role I want you to assume and play is this: you recreate, and bring alive in your mind, the anxiety, the stiff neck and the palpitations along with the lack of motivation, the negative feelings, emptiness and purposelessness. I want you to try and experience them in all their negative emotional load. Do this recreation in a way that if somebody sees you, he/she thinks that you are really experiencing unbearable anxiety, concern and negative feelings. If you manage to do the exercise as I have instructed you to, we will get the best outcomes. There is the possibility that you make the best effort, but you cannot make the role resemble the actual experience by 100%. As long as you do your best, it doesn't matter how close it is to the actual experience. There may be times when you make the effort, but you fail to conjure up those states of mind completely. This is still okay. You may also forget to do the exercise on time, or you may be outside or with a friend, or fail to do the exercise for any reasons. If this happens, you lost the opportunity to do that exercise and you cannot make up for it. You simply wait for the next exercise time. In other words, you either don't do the exercise, or you do it on time. I need to give me two times that fit into your daily schedule, so that you can do the exercises then.

C: 18:00 and 23:00.

T: The important thing is that you should start tomorrow, not today. Also, doing these exercises doesn't mean that you are not allowed to have the anxiety and the negative thoughts and emotions. You know very well that they are beyond your control, and invade your mind without you asking for them. The only thing within your control is the exercise that you must do twice a day according to the instructions I gave you. You don't do anything to deal with the anxiety at other times of the day. You don't decide or think anything. They may either come to you or not. Next session, we can talk about what happened.

Session Two

T: Welcome back. Tell me what you did.

C: I didn't manage to do the exercise regularly, at first. But I gradually got better and did them all right. I can say that I have been able to pull myself together, as a result of doing the exercises. I have more self-confidence and self-assurance.

T: Before we talk more about the self-assurance, let me ask you this: what happened to the anxiety and the negative feelings during the past two weeks?

C: It was interesting to me that, during the exercises, I was able to recreate the emotions only once or twice. I couldn't conjure them no matter how hard I tried. In general, I felt really good. I don't know why. I guess it was because the university agreed for me to continue my studies, which was a great news and lifted the pressure from me. I have also decreased my medication. I take drugs three times a day.

T: You said that you have self-assurance. What are its signs?

C: I was able to do things. I did the work I've been delaying for a long time.

T: How about the lack of motivation, emptiness and purposelessness?

C: I think the lack of motivation was with me during the last two weeks, and presented itself in the form of escaping from reality. During the last two weeks, I realized that I escaped reality a lot.

T: How do you sleep, now?

C: Better than before. There are times when I can't go to sleep out of fear. But there were also times when I was able to sleep soundly, and I didn't have to wake up to have drugs.

T: In general, I think that you have made some progress. As for the rest of our work, I believe you should keep on doing the exercises as good as before, or even better, so that you can stop your medication after the next session. Taking into account your own condition, maybe you can decrease it further and omit it altogether by the time we will have our next session. Do the exercises twice a day (19:00 and 23:00), each time for 5 min.

Session Three

T: Welcome back. We were supposed to meet in two weeks, but you were busy and couldn't make it. It's been six weeks since we had our last session together. Please, tell me what you did.

C: I'm sorry I couldn't come along and missed a therapy session. I did the exercises during the first two weeks, but then I had to go on a trip. I couldn't do them in the meantime. Last week, when I came back, I started doing them again.

T: And how have you been?

C: I feel much better. I did my best during the first two weeks to do the exercises completely. The results were similar to those of the session before that. I was able to do things, I slept soundly, and the anxiety and lack of motivation have decreased. I didn't feel those negative states of mind for some time. And I have decreased my medication to one or two a day. I feel much better, in general.

T: Thank you for doing the exercises. Well, there was a journey that prevented you from doing the exercises completely, and you couldn't make an appointment any sooner. At the same time, your report today shows that you've been making progress. Since we have summer holidays ahead of us, I can't draw a new timetable for you, and you'd better stick to your present schedule and make the changes I will point out, until September when we can have another session. You do your best to decrease the medication and finally stop it completely. Do the exercise for the previous session (two 5-min exercises at 19:00 and 23:00) for one more week. As for the week after that, do the same exercise just on even days. Then, stop doing the exercises till September.

Session Four

T: Welcome back. We had the summer break after our last session together. We were supposed to resume your treatment in September, but you didn't come back till now, which makes it 18 months. Please, tell me what you did, and how you are now.

C: I tried to stop my medication, as you instructed me to, and I succeeded. It's been months now that I take one pill a month. Although I know that 1 pill won't have any effects during a whole month, I still can't give it up.

T: Just take that 1 pill, because it's no big deal and you mustn't bother yourself over it. How about your other issues?

C: Since 6 months ago, I've been experiencing lack of motivation again. I have lost all hope, and I don't care about my life and the future. There are times when I wish the world comes to an end and it's all over. The center of all the hopelessness and lack of motivation is my educational failure. I always wished to have a scientific career. But I look at myself now and see someone with an average of 12 who is barely getting his BA. I feel I have lost everything and it's all gone. Then, I don't care about job, marriage or anything else. Despite all this, I didn't resume medication, except for that one pill a month.

T: You said, previously, that you felt like there were two aspects, or two persons, in you. Whatever one built, the other one destroyed. It was an important issue with you, which we intended to deal with after getting over your anxiety and lack of motivation. Let me tell you something about this duality, and then we can get to your new exercises. Look! The basis of all your problems is the situation the destroyer has caused for the builder. The destroyer is not harmful, just because he waits for things to be built so he can destroy them. He has a more fundamental function which makes him the winner all the time. He has been able to influence the mindset and the decisions of the builder, making him set one and only one goal for himself: a very ambitious one. He has been able to make the builder adopt the wrong decision and has made him believe that he must have only this one goal. In the meantime, he has made the goal seem so valuable that the builder cannot be satisfied with any other goals. Why? Because the builder will be totally vulnerable and can be defeated in the battle against the destroyer. If a person is able to define a set of goals for himself, when he fails to attain one of them, he turns to another one rather than thinking the world has come to an end. The destroyer has been able to delude the builder in this way, and that is why the builder always fails. We must change this formula. This is the target we are following at this stage of the treatment.[1]

After you have had your exam next week, do the following exercise. Divide your days into evens (Saturday, Monday and Wednesday) and odds (Sunday, Tuesday and Thursday). Odd days are for the destroyer, while even days belong to the builder. On odd days, all your feelings, emotions, actions, decisions and plans are arranged by the bad guy. And on even days they are all defined by the good guy. On odd days, you try to be hopeless, unmotivated, negative and full of bad feelings, just as the destroyer wants. Do whatever he has been doing over the years to wreck your life. On even days, you do your best to set goals, be hopeful and motivated, see things in a positive light and have good feelings. You are free on Fridays, and you mustn't assume either the role of the destroyer or that of the builder.[2]

Session Five

T: It is nice to meet you again. Tell me what you did.

C: I did my best, but it was difficult for me to assume the role of the destroyer or the builder throughout a whole day. I spent a large part of the day in university, at class or with my friends, where I couldn't play the role. I did try to do the exercise at times I was alone. Also, when I was happy and contented during the day, I could no longer play the role of the destroyer. Because my mood was against the role. On even days, when I was supposed to play the role of the builder, it was good and nothing went wrong. But, on odd days, when I was supposed to play the role of the destroyer, I couldn't make it bad enough, and sometimes I got the opposite result.

T: Thank you for your report. I have a general idea, now, of what you did. How do you evaluate your own work? How did you feel in general?

C: I wanted everything to be good. I felt good during the two weeks, and I didn't like to assume negative roles.

T: I understand your desire to be good, and it's great to hear that you have been much better during the last two weeks. But what I want to know is that you manage to play the role of the destroyer to some extent. What were the differences between this role, and the actual destroyer who takes control and wrecks everything?

C: The difference was that when I played his role, there was no trace of the negative feelings and the lost hopes and the subsequent bad mood. Before this, it had a really negative influence on me, and made me feel really bad for some time.

T: I think it's been a great experience, and you have done your duty during the exercises. The instruction for you is to feel commitment to do the exercises. It is okay if you forget to do it, or fail to do it for any reasons, or manage to do only 30 to 40% of your daily exercises. Keep on doing the same exercise up to the next session. Play the role of the destroyer on odd days, and that of the builder on even days, as much as you get the chance.

Session Six

T: Welcome back. Did you do your exercises?

C: I went home during this time, and I spent most of my time with family. Due to my own condition, when I used to go back home, I didn't feel well. This time, however, it was great. I worked hard on even days, and on odd days, I couldn't assume the role of the destroyer no

[1] The PTC model does not require giving such explanations and analyses. In other words, the paradoxical timetable is a perfect and comprehensive technique that can deal with any problems on itself. Such analyses serve an inspiring purpose and increase the client's understanding of the process of treatment, thereby encouraging his/her cooperation. Therefore, the PTC therapist can either adopt, or let go of, such analyses based on the client's level of understanding, motivation and preparedness.

[2] You can learn more about this paradoxical technique, called "the turn-taking management timetable" in *PTC perfect model of therapy with couples: A practical guide* (Besharat 2018).

matter how I tried. It has become difficult for me to have negative feelings or play negative roles. I was also able to take care of a lot of stuff I'd been delaying for a long time. So, I am really satisfied.

T: How were you when you went back to the university?

C: I came back last week. The good mood has been with me here, too. It is difficult for me to play the negative role, here, as well.

T: Taking into account your experience, how do you evaluate your general mood from the beginning of our sessions together up to now?

C: Right now, I am in a great mood and I am contented. It's been some time now that I've been following my goals, and there isn't anybody or anything that can destroy them or disturb me. The destroyer hasn't been able to take control of me, destroy what I have built and defeat me. I think that is why I've been able to take care of my life and live with hope and positive feelings. I'm just worried whether this good condition will prevail or not.

T: We have now reached our therapeutic goals. However, we have to wait to see what happens in the future. Will your good condition prevail? In my opinion, it is possible that your improvement and treatment will prevail by more than 90%. What you did through the sessions was to empower the good guy, so that he wouldn't have to give in to the bad guy and be defeated. You did this important job, and you are no longer after of the bad guy and his pressure and presence. It's been some time since you've started being active and taking control of your life. In future, anytime that upsetting situation presents itself, you can adopt the same method for dealing with it so as to turn the table to your advantage and not give in. Right now, you have so much power and authority that you can't bring the bad guy back although you try. Formerly, you didn't want the bad guy to come to you, but he came anyway.

This is our last session together. You continue doing the exercises for two more weeks, at the maximum. Then, live your normal life. If your problem emerges again in the future, wait for a number of days in order to make sure that the bad guy is back for good. Then, draw a similar timetable for yourself and stick to it. You will definitely get the same outcome, and you will regain control. In any case, I'd be glad to see you again if you feel the need to see me. Good luck!

19.3 Assessment of Treatment Outcome and Follow-Up

The course of the treatment was completed in 6 sessions. Assessment of the treatment outcome, which was based on the patients' comments in a graded scale of 0–100 and an open-ended question, indicated 100% recovery. A 2-month follow-up evaluation showed no relapse.

20 Client #18 (Female, 27 Years Old, Divorced)

20.1 Case Introduction

Mrs. SY, a 27-year-old woman, came to the University of Tehran Clinic complaining about negative thoughts and obsessions, self-blaming and feeling guilty. She got married 5 years ago and divorced after 2 years. SY is now living with her parents. It's more than 5 months that her problems got much worse with a clinical depression ending. She presented with serious distress and symptoms of clinical depression: "I have no motivation. I just want to die. If it weren't for my religious beliefs, I would have committed suicide. I feel like dying. I want something happen to me and kill me". SY has also been suffering social anxiety disorder and fear of driving since years ago. The clinical interview based on DSM-5 (APA 2013), revealed that SY had the criteria for both major depressive disorder and social anxiety disorder. All these resulted in serious problems for SY's in her study and interpersonal relationships, specifically with her family members. YS has received several psychiatric and psychological treatments with no improvement of her clinical condition before coming to our clinic. SY was seen for 6 sessions over a period of 11 weeks.

20.2 Course of Treatment

Session One

Therapist (T): (After greetings and the social stage of the interview) Tell me why you are here, please.

Client (C): I am devastated. I have so many problems, I don't know where to start.

T: We have enough time for you to talk about all of them. You can tell me about the one that's been bothering you more than others, or start from anywhere you like.

C: I have lost my power of judgment since four months ago. Whatever I do and whatever I say, I think I have made a mistake seconds later. I keep criticizing myself. It's gotten worse. I say something to someone in the office. Then I tell my sister, "that was a stupid thing to say." "What did you say?" my sister asks. And when I tell her what I've said, she says what I've said is correct and reasonable. I have lost the criteria for good and bad, and right and wrong. And I know the reason. It's because I've been divorced. I always rebuke myself.

T: When were you divorced?

C: It's been two years and a half.

T: How long were you married?

C: Two years.

T: Why did you get divorced?

C: I filed for divorce myself. We both agreed to get divorced. My husband suffered from a severe mental illness. I regretted it right after I got married. I rebuked myself so much, because my family had warned me. I didn't listen! (She offers a thorough account of her marriage and divorce).

T: You said that you've lost your power of judgment since four months ago. What else?

M. A. Besharat, *Paradoxical Psychotherapy: A Practitioner's Guide*, University of Tehran Science and Humanities Series,
https://doi.org/10.1007/978-3-031-27717-7_20

C: I see myself banging on my head with a large hammer or an axe. I just keep hitting my head with them. I see the image so clearly (starts crying). I have lost my self-confidence. If someone criticizes me, I'm like "Look? She sees how stupid you are, too." I want to learn a new language, and I can't. Then, I think this is because I am incompetent. I keep looking for ways to prove to myself that I am incapable. Really incapable! All these have made me lose my motivation. I have no motivation. I just want to die. If it weren't for my religious beliefs, I would have committed suicide. I feel like dying. I want something happen to me and kill me.

T: How long have you been like this?

C: I have always been like this, more or less. But it got worse four to five months ago, and never left me alone. I keep reprimanding myself and I can't get a break. I see myself guilty of everything. After my divorce, my family was so upset. My father was broken. Whenever I see him, I am upset. I feel I am guilty.

T: What have you done so far to solve your problem? From personal arrangements to visiting a specialist?

C: I talked about my problems with some people. They said I was the one who must help myself. So I reached the decision that nobody could help me. And I can't myself or do anything about it. I felt worse as time went by. I visited specialists twice or three times. But it didn't work (gives explanations about her previous visits to specialists).

T: Well, it's my turn now. We need to have several sessions together. I prescribe for you some exercises that you need to do in the interval between the sessions. Just, keep in mind that as long as you are receiving my treatment, you cannot go to any other specialist or do anything on your own. You must let my treatment to be completed and don't interrupt it with your or others' interventions.

All these negative thoughts and obsessions have overwhelmed you now and don't allow you to think clearly, to make good judgments or analyses or to live. First, we need to give you back the control of your life. When this happens you can, like everyone else, think, decide and act correctly. Here's what I want you to do: you find a calm place where nobody or nothing can disrupt you and you can focus on your task. You try and recreate the bitter memories of all the sexual violence (experience in the relationship with her husband), and re-experience them as if they are happening to you then and there. You need to make this second-hand experience just as disturbing, upsetting and moving as the original experiences. For the first three days, do this twice a day for 10 min. From the fourth day up to our next session together, do it once a day. This time, try to recreate and re-experience negative thoughts and feelings about yourself. Think that you are stupid, incompetent, helpless and guilty. You need to make an honest and real effort to make the exercise identical with the actual feelings and experiences you've had. If this happens, it is perfect and you will get the best outcome. However, there is a possibility that despite your honest effort, you fail to recreate the original mood and succeed by just 50%. As long as you make your best effort, it doesn't matter. There is also a possibility that you can conjure zero negative memories and fail altogether in your endeavor. This is still okay, since you have done your duty. There is also another possibility. Let's say you are supposed to do exercise at 10, but you oversleep, forget, are with a friend or are outside at that time. So you can't do the exercise. In this case, if you fail to do the exercise on time, you should let it go and mustn't try to make up for it. You just wait for the next turn of the exercise. The reason is that you either don't do these exercises, or you do them exactly on time. Now, you give me two times according to daily schedule, when you are most likely to be free in order to do the exercises. Also, you must start doing the exercises tomorrow, not today.

C: 14:00 and 23:00 are fine.

T: From the fourth day on, do the first exercise at 14:00 and the second one at 23:00. There is one more point. The only thing you need to do about your problem is to do the exercises regularly. You shouldn't do anything else. You can't go to other specialists. You can't do anything on your own so as to make yourself feel better. No! You won't do anything. You won't think anything and you won't decide anything. Forget about other times of the day. Whatever happens, we can talk about it the next session.

Session Two

T: Nice to see you again. Tell me what you did with the exercises.

C: I managed to do the exercises well. Every time I did it, the memories came rushing back and I couldn't stop crying. I got goose bumps. After a couple of times, however, it got less intense. As for the second exercise, I was supposed to recreate my broodings and thoughts. I couldn't do it at first. They came, but they didn't make me upset like they always do. They were mainly artificial. I couldn't concentrate my thoughts.

T: What else?

C: I forgot to mention something last session. I used to drive. I was a good driver and everything was fine. When I was married, my husband kept finding fault with my driving, and I couldn't drive after that. I can't even sit behind the wheels of a parked car. Our car is in the parking and no body uses it. My parents keep asking me to drive, but I can't.

T: What do you think will happen if you drive a car?

C: I'm afraid that if I start driving, and someone says something to me, I can't go on driving anymore. Or that the car goes off and I can't switch it on again.

T: Did you say you were a good driver before?

C: Yes, I was really good. I got my license when I was 18 and I drove our car for years.

T: How long has it been since you last drove a car?

C: It's been six years. There is also something else. The way my father treats me really bothers me. My father is old, and he tries to be kind and good to me at home. But I get really angry and I want to throw something at him. It's so annoying! He is a great and caring father. I don't know why I treat him that way. I can't control my behavior, no matter how I try.

T: Is there anything else?

C: When I have to give speeches, I'm scared out of my wits. My body starts trembling. My mouth goes all dry. It is so stressful for me. I have to give a speech in two weeks, and I'm afraid of it right now.

T: How often do you meet your father?

C: Just during weekends when I'm home.

T: So, we have your father, driving and giving speeches. You have had a good start with your exercises. Let's see how we can move on. Let's deal with the driving problem later on, because your father and your speech are priorities. Keep on doing the two previous exercises twice for 10 min. For the first week, start with imagine bitter memories and end with demeaning thoughts about yourself (C: At 18"00). During the first week, do another 10-min exercise about your father. Imagine that your father wants to caress you, say kind words to you or do anything that makes you angry, and you feel that you want to throw something at him. Imagine that your father has done whatever it is he does, and you have reacted angrily (C: At 14:00 and 23:00). Do these exercises up to the end of the week when you go home to your father and mother. When you come back the next week, you must do two 10-min exercises a day about your conference (C: At 14:00 and 23:00). Imagine that the conference has come, your body is trembling, your mouth is dry, you have panicked and you humiliate yourself with a disastrous speech. Since the conference is held after our next session, I will tell you what to do on the day of the conference, then. Also, do a 5-min exercise following the previous one, about your bitter sexual experience and the negative thoughts (C: At 18:00).

Session Three

T: It's nice to see you again. Please tell me what you did.

C: Doing the exercise about my father was really difficult. I need to explain something here. Right after my divorce, I curse at God and the prophet in my mind. I always did it up to a few months ago. I hit myself and curse at myself. I swore at myself loudly. I did this so that the voice in my mind would stop, but it wouldn't. It was the worst when I needed to concentrate and study. After a while, it stopped and didn't happen again. I thought you may need to know this.

T: All right! So what happened in the exercise about your father?

C: Whenever I did this exercise, I hated myself. It wasn't like this with other exercises about the negative thoughts and the sexual relationship. But after that exercise, I felt hatred for myself. This is why it was difficult for me. And I had guests over at my place, so I couldn't do some of the exercises.

T: Did you go home during the weekend?

C: Yes.

T: What happened?

C: It was worse.

T: Do you mean your feelings toward your father had become worse?

C: Yes.

T: What about the conference?

C: Actually, I couldn't do that exercise well enough.

T: What about the exercise of thoughts and experiences?

C: It's really interesting. During the first two weeks, I cried bitterly whenever I did those exercises. I got goose bumps. During the last two weeks, however, I didn't cry and have goose bumps at all. The memories are not bitter to me, anymore. I had a dream after a long time. I dreamed I'd gotten married and had sexual intercourse. I reached orgasm. It was a sweet dream.

T: You have had a good and valuable experience. The emotional load of the bitter sexual experience you've had is no longer there. You have been able to have a dream about a satisfying sexual intercourse. It tells you and me that our method has been effective. Since I believe that the basis of all your problems is the same, continuing the exercises can help you with your other problems as well. I said this because I want you to be aware of the work you are doing and do the rest of the exercises more carefully. Don't lose the chance of doing the exercises easily. The more you can do the exercises and spend time and energy on them, the faster you will have the favorable outcomes. When do you have to give a presentation, tomorrow?

C: At 10:00.

T: Do the exercise about the conference tonight and tomorrow morning (C: At 23:00 and 6:00) as I've already instructed you to. Tomorrow, at the university and before going to give your speech, you mustn't think, wish or pray, under any circumstances, that you have a good speech. No! You must go to the conference with the expectation that you will do really bad on your speech. If you let any other thoughts enter your mind, you won't get the proper results. Think and act just as I've instructed you to. Since you are not going to have another speech till the next session, we don't have anything to do with it anymore. I'll receive your report on it next session, and make decisions. Keep on doing the exercises about your father twice a day, for 10 min, according to my instruction (C: At 14:00 and 23:00). See you next session.

Session Four

T: Welcome back. Tell me what you did, please.

C: I did really well on my speech. I didn't have the anxiety I was scared of. I had a bottle of water with me, but my mouth wasn't dry at all. I didn't feel hot. I just couldn't look at my friends. I had everything under control and did really well. My friends were like "you did really well, you just didn't look at us." I did well.

T: Well, that's a step forward. You didn't have enough time to do the exercises. In future, we will make plans so you can have more time to exercise. I remember you saying that you have no more speeches till the end of the term. Yet, you do have the counselor-client role-playing task in your class. When is it due?

C: I have to announce a time myself, which I still haven't. Now, I think that I'm not scared of it as much as I used to.

T: We will make a timetable for you at the end of the session. How did you do with the exercise about your father?

C: I did my best to do the exercises, and I managed to do them better than before. At first, I felt great anger at my father. But gradually, the anger went away. I'd become indifferent toward it. When I went home during the weekend, I felt much better toward my father.

I told you about my dream, last session. It was a long time I had forgotten about sexual pleasure. After that dream, however, I felt like my sexual desire is activated. On the one hand, I'm happy since it makes me energetic and enthusiastic. On the other hand, I'm afraid it might hurt my studies. I have a great sexual desire and when it is active, it's really difficult for me to control it. That's why I decided to get married so soon. I'm afraid it may cause problems for me again.

T: This experience and the stimulation of your sexual desire is good and positive. It both shows that you have gone through constructive changes. It is an indication of happiness and enthusiasm. It shows that the inhibition and suppression of this desire are no longer there. I don't think you need to suppress this desire. Because it shows that you are alive. You must manage and direct it so that doesn't cause you problems. Don't worry about how to control this desire. Let it flow freely for the time being. I can help you control it later on, if it is necessary. What else?

C: That's all.

T: I think we are doing well. Your report shows that good things are happening with your father. What you told me was, in my opinion, positive. One purpose was that this daughter shouldn't feel guilty toward her father anymore. This has begun, and we are on the right track. What is going to happen next? What kind of emotion will take the place of anger and guilt? The same emotion most people feel toward their elderly fathers. Most people feel respect and kindness for their fathers. This doesn't mean, however, that old age is fun and enjoyable. Quite the reverse. When children see how old and infirm their parents have become, they are upset. One should both deal with the problems of old age, and treat the elderly well. But, no one should feel guilt. You should now do a 10-min exercise about your father every day (C: At 8:30). Recreate and re-experience any hatred, anger, spite and negative feelings you have for your father. You said something about the exercises which weren't part of my instructions for you. During the exercises, don't talk! Just do the exercise! You added some analyses to the exercises, which isn't right. You are not allowed to analyze anything while doing the exercises. You told yourself that your father is old and you have to respect him, and all that. Don't tell yourself such things during the exercises I have ordered you to do! You need to do two exercises for the counselor-client role-playing task. Imagine, within two 10-min sessions that have ruined the task. The class laughs at you and criticizes you. You can't deal with the task and it is a disaster. Imagine all the worst things happening to you during the task. (C: At 14:00 and 23:00) See you next session.

Session Five

T: Nice to see you again. Tell me what you did.

C: I had to do two exercises, one about my father and the other one about the fear of role-playing in class. I did the exercises and I'm so satisfied. This time, when I went home, I didn't feel angry at my father at all. I have changed so much.

T: Can we say that you feel less bad about father?

C: I don't feel bad at all. I understand him.

T: What about the role-playing in the class? Did you get a chance to do it?

C: The professor changed the schedule. I guess I'll do my turn tomorrow. But I'm not afraid of doing it anymore, and I know I'll do it fine.

T: What else?

C: Last session, I said that I feel alive and I have sexual desire, but I'm afraid of it. I don't know whether I can deal with them, or you need to make an intervention. I've been a lot better since three weeks ago. I'm not preoccupied with sexual fantasies that take so much of my time (like before my marriage), and I feel good. I don't know if I have gained control over it, or whether my sexual desire is not fully activated yet.

T: What about negative feelings about bitter past experience, and brooding over your personal worth?

C: They have decreased greatly. They come and immediately go. They no longer stick in my mind to torture me. Also, I feel self-confident, now, and I know that I can deal with them if they come. They don't exert control over me anymore.

T: That's great.

C: I feel it's a miracle. Others tell me "you look happy. You look so different." I feel the same way. I enjoy my life, now. There is just this thing that has been with me since childhood, and is really annoying. I avoid the things I have to do. I postpone them. For instance, I have to study the English language, and I keep coming up with these excuses so as not to do it.

T: Were you like this since childhood?

C: Yes, but it has become annoying now. Now that my other problems have been solved, I would like to deal with this problem too.

T: Yes, we can deal with that too. However, this characteristic has a different nature from the problems we have dealt with so far. That is probably why you preferred to discuss the other problems first. We should wait a little bit, so that your treatment is complete. Then, we can begin working on this new problem.

So far, negative thoughts about yourself, bitter past memories, tension of a more or less sexual nature, conflict with the father and the anxiety of talking to a crowd (class) have been resolved. We have to give them time to be over for good. And we also need to deal with the fear of driving. We will probably have two more sessions so as for the treatment to be completed. Then, three to six months must pass before we can begin a new treatment process for that say personality trait you talked about. We may not need to deal with it, however, since it may be resolved on its own as your present problems are solved. As long as that personality trait has been influenced by your other problems, it would go away.

You said that you will probably have the councilor-client role-playing task in class, tomorrow and you will tell me about the results next session. Until next session, I will draw you a timetable about your fear of driving. Your task is this: for the first week, two 10-min exercises when you imagine the worst that could happen to you while driving. The engine goes dead, others make fun of you, you have an accident, you are stuck in traffic, you panic and whatever else that can be upsetting to you. The instruction for this exercise is the same as before, and I think you've done it so much we can consider it as your internship. For the second week, you must do the two 10-min exercises in the car. You get into the car, sit behind the wheels, and do the exercise. You don't switch the car on. After three days, you will be ready to turn the car on and drive. Where you go and what you do depends on how feel then. You may want to switch the car on and off. You may prefer to move around the parking. You may move outside at a time when streets are empty and drive around. Your mood at the time can tell you what to do exactly.

C: Doctor! Do I need to recreate my ex-husband's rebukes and disagreements?

T: Thanks for reminding me. Yes you do, because it's related to your fear of driving.

Session Six

T: Welcome back. Tell me what you did.

C: (offering cookies to the therapist) This is for my driving.

T: Thank you. So, you did it?

C: Yes. I couldn't believe it. I went with my brother, and I drove easily.

T: Did you do the exercises?

C: I did. The exercises themselves were no problem. But getting prepared to do the exercise was a little difficult. It was as if something held me back to not go and do the exercise. When I started, however, it was easy to do. It was the same the first time I wanted to get in the car. I wanted to escape. But the second I entered the car, it was over. I didn't even need to just sit in the car and do the exercise for three days. The first time I entered the car, I felt that I'm ready to drive.

T: All right. Problem solved. Last session, you mentioned the sexual desire and how it's active now, and you said that you were worried. I wanted first to deal with your stress and the fear of driving, as the last traces of your anxiety, and then give it some time to see what happens to the desire. We can deal with it in this session.

C: Doctor, within the last two years, after my divorce, I didn't have any relationships, and I didn't want any. I had many suitors, but I didn't want to get married. I had another suitor last week. Our families arranged it. My family wanted me to talk to him. But you had said that we must first deal with my problems. Is this the right time? Am I ready for it? What do you say I should do?

T: First tell me about your sexual desire.

C: It has increased a lot.

T: Is it pleasurable for you?

C: Yes, and it's not annoying at all, which is interesting to me. It was annoying to me before. I was worried that it might be the same this time, as well. But no! It's not annoying at all. It's quite fulfilling and I would like to be able to get married soon, and have babies. But I'm afraid.

T: Because of your former experience, or what?

C: Both my family and I want me to get married soon. Also, I'm driven by sexual desire and need. So, I'm afraid that I might not be able to see everything and make a mistake again like last time. That is why I'm not sure whether I am ready to talk to suitors and make decisions or not.

T: Have you ever tried, on your own, to satisfy your sexual need, after it has been activated again?

C: No. Sometimes, I feel the need during the day. My body beats like a pulse. I hadn't experienced something like this for a long time. But I have never done anything.

(Sex therapy techniques were adopted to resolve this issue and concern.) Now, let's review everything one more time. The negative thoughts, broodings, and the father?

C: I am much better. Relationship with my father is not 100% good. But, it's a lot better. I have higher tolerance and less guilty feelings.

T: Under such circumstances, this improvement and change is good enough. How about thoughts of yourself? And the role-playing task?

C: Last week, I played the role of counselor before the class, and it was fine. The professor and the students criticized me a lot, and I got really angry. It was annoying, but I immediately felt better. It was like a real experience for me. My main problem was appearing before a crowd and giving a presentation. I was able to do it without any anxiety.

T: So, you can appear before a crowd (class). Hearing criticism and reacting to it is about personal differences, and it's not a problem per se. Are you like this only in class, or everywhere?

C: It's everywhere. For example, when I enter a wedding, I stare at the ground and go sit somewhere. Everyone thinks how rude I am, but it's actually because of anxiety. I have difficulty in formal meetings. At times, I've tried to mingle in, so as to deal with my fear. But it didn't help.

T: You can have some exercises in this regard. When you leave here, do two 10-min exercises (C: At 14:30 and 22:30) every day for the first two weeks, one exercise a day (C: At 2:30) for the third week and on even days (C: At 22:30) for the fourth week until your problem is solved. You must recreate all the related scenes in these exercises: entering a wedding ceremony, giving a speech at a conference and entering the class or a formal meeting. And in all these places, everyone stares at you. You become red in the face and you get tremor. You feel awkward while saying hello. You must re-imagine and re-experience all these annoying and humiliating thoughts and feelings. When you are actually in the situation (similar to the speech given at the conference), you must tell yourself that the worst will happen. While doing the exercises, if the change for appearing in a real life situation—a wedding ceremony for example—shows up, you must change your exercise accordingly. Do for the wedding ceremony all that you did for the conference. You will definitely succeed in dealing with this problem, too. You have already made good progress in this regard, as the conference and the role-playing experience suggest. But you will get better. I will be available in the future, anytime you need me.

20.3 Assessment of Treatment Outcome and Follow-Up

The course of the treatment was completed in 6 sessions. Assessment of the treatment outcome, which was based on the patients' comments in a graded scale of 0–100 and an open-ended question, indicated 100% recovery. A three-year follow-up evaluation revealed no relapse.

21 Client #19 (Male, 26 Years Old, Single)

21.1 Case Introduction

Mr. KA, a 26-year-old student, was referred to the University of Tehran Clinic because of his serious OCD symptoms. He developed his symptoms as becoming paranoid about his two younger brothers, showing no concern about his appearance, increased sexual desire, meanwhile presenting depressive mood and losing weight at age 18. The symptoms gradually changed to more as obsessive and compulsive disorder rather than a pure psychotic one as shown at the beginning. He has been under psychiatric care taking medications for more than 4 years continuously with just a very little improvement on his depressive symptoms. The clinical interview based on DSM-5 (APA 2013), confirmed KA's OCD. KA's clinical condition had a great impact on his relationships with others including his family. He is now living at a university dormitory and is at a great risk of being expelled from college. This is his first visit to receive a psychological treatment. KA was seen for 4 sessions over a period of 5 weeks.

21.2 Course of Treatment

Session One

Therapist (T): (After greetings and the social stage of the interview) Please tell me why you are here.

Client (C): My two younger brothers and I used to live in the same room. It was about eight years ago when I was studying for the university entrance exam. One night, I saw one of my brothers motioned to the other and they both went outside to study. Suddenly, this event sparked off a whole chain of sensitivity in my mind, and my confusion started. From then on, all my attention went to them and I lost focus for studying.

T: Your problem started eight years ago before the university entrance exam when you became sensitive about your two brothers. How did you feel?

C: I hated it when they were together; not that I was suspicious they were talking about me. I just didn't like it. My mind always turned to them and I wondered what they might be doing together, and why they are together, and I couldn't start studying unless they separated. For two months, I felt like this only about my two brothers. After that, my feeling extended to others. From then on, any two people who are together attract my mind and my attention.

T: What quality does this mental preoccupation with couples have? Is it good, bad, pleasant or unpleasant?

C: It's unpleasant, since it prevents me from focusing on my work.

T: What do they do when they enter your mind?

C: I imagined them sitting down and talking, and spending time together. It wasn't suspicion,

M. A. Besharat, *Paradoxical Psychotherapy: A Practitioner's Guide*,
University of Tehran Science and Humanities Series,
https://doi.org/10.1007/978-3-031-27717-7_21

since they were my brothers and I loved them, but I didn't like the fact that they were together. After a month, I couldn't sleep anymore and I lost more than 20 kg. I felt great stress. Nevertheless, I succeeded in the exam since I had studied hard, and I entered university. The problem has been with me ever since, though. It got so bad that I lost any motivation. I didn't care how I look; I didn't like anything; I didn't care whether I was clean or not; sometimes I wore dirty, ragged clothes. I'd become so sloppy.

T: You mean you didn't care about your appearance, your clothes or your personal hygiene?

C: I didn't care at all. My friends said, a university student isn't supposed to look like that. They didn't understand what I was going through.

T: So, you suffered from this problem, and you couldn't sleep well; what about your eating?

C: I ate well. I brood over things a lot. For example, I pick up a book to study, and I feel that all the people are talking about me. They say "he's become a bum, he has given up his studies." They don't know about my problem. Even my mother thought that I was lying and there was no problem with me. I took her to my psychiatrist once, so he could tell her about my problem. The doctor explained my problem to her. But she still didn't believe it that much.

T: Did you say your obsession extended to others later on?

C: Yes, I felt it about any two people who were together. For example, before my turn came up, two people were here with you. My mind was totally preoccupied with them. There always has to be something preoccupying my mind. When there is no body for me to obsess over, the things around me attract my attention; like the ashtray, the picture on the wall, the watch or something. When I take something away so I wouldn't have to look at it all the time, something else enters my mind. It's impossible for my mind to remain completely focused on my lessons.

T: You said you couldn't sleep but you ate well. Can you remember how your sexual desire was?

C: It had increased a lot. I was under a lot of pressure in this regard. I am not an immoral person, but my sexual desire had increased so much that I constantly ejaculated in my sleep. Now, when I look at a woman in the street, I see her naked. When I go to bed, I imagine that the woman is beside me naked. I have these thoughts about by close relatives as well. Sometimes they are so close I am ashamed to tell you who they are.

T: So, when you look at women related to you and other women in the streets, you see them naked and you are sexually aroused, right?

C: Yes.

T: Your imagination has to be very fertile to be able to see them naked.

C: Exactly! For example, this happens when I see women in family parties. I leave the party, go outside and cry; because I am a religious person and always say my prayers.

T: What kind of treatments have you received for your problem?

C: I have seen many psychiatrists. It's been four years since I started taking drugs. The last psychiatrist has told me that if I don't get well in a month (which will make it 18 months since I started taking his prescribed medication), I have to be hospitalized.

T: How have these drugs helped you so far?

C: They didn't help at all. I've been taking drugs for years, and it's all been useless.

T: You said that there has to be something in your mind, and you gave the example of the watch, and the picture on the wall. Now, do you like them to come to your mind, or do they come for themselves?

C: They come for themselves. I hate to think about them, since they interrupt me and prevent me from studying.

T: Do you have any problems other than these thoughts, and the sexual fantasies?

C: There isn't anything else.

T: You said that you didn't care about your appearance and personal hygiene during a period. What about now?

C: I've become better in this respect.

T: How do you sleep?

C: My sleep has become better as well.

T: Your current psychiatrist has told you that if the medication doesn't treat you within the last month, you must be hospitalized. Do you think the medication will help you during this month?

C: Not at all. I have no doubt that no good will come of them within this last month.

T: I agree with you on that. The medication won't change anything within the last month. If drugs were going to be helpful at all, they would have treated you in the past four years and you would have felt some change and improvement. So, you should consider stopping the medication. You can either consult your psychiatrist or, if you have ceased taking medication before, just decide on your own. Either way, it's better for you to stop the medication as soon as possible. I will arrange a different treatment plan for you here. If you stick to this treatment, and follow my instructions, you can be treated without any drugs.

According to this new treatment, you must do certain tasks or exercises as I instruct you to. To do this exercise, you must set aside 10 min and find a place where you can focus and not be disrupted by anybody or anything. You will allot the first half of these 10 min to recreating thoughts and worries about couples, and during the second half, you recreate thoughts about things. What I mean by recreating thoughts and worries about couples is that you must try, during the exercise, to bring to your mind voluntarily the thoughts and worries that preoccupy your mind unintentionally and bother you. You must make the conscious effort to summon to your mind those disturbing worries and thoughts with all the stress and pressure accompanying them, to the extent that you start feeling really upset and uneasy. The same thing is true about things as well; just like when thoughts about things enter your mind and prevent you from focusing and studying, you must try to bring them to your mind and re-experience them and the discomfort and agitation attached to them. When you sit down to do the exercise, one of the following possibilities might present itself: you might be able to recreate the thoughts and worries with all the distress and anxiety aroused by them, just as I have instructed you to do. If this happens, we will get the best outcomes. There is however, the possibility that you only manage by 50%, despite your honest effort. If this happens, you don't need to worry as long as you've given it your best shot. You might make an effort but you cannot recreate any thoughts at all during the 10 min. In other words, the recreation is zero. It's again okay, as long as you make your best endeavor. There is also the possibility that you miss a session because you oversleep, or you are outside, or you are not alone, or whatever. You fail to do the task right on time. In this case, the exercise is lost and you are not allowed to do make up for it at some other time. You either do these tasks and exercises precisely on time, or you don't do them at all. So, that is what you are supposed to do. Now, I need you to give me two times during the day when you can do the task for 10 min.

C: I can do it at 7:00 and 19:00.

T: Starting from tomorrow, your task is to do the exercise at these two times just as I instructed you. Pay attention that all I am asking you is to do the exercise according to the timetables we have agreed on. I don't ask you to do anything else. I don't want you to do anything special at other times of the day. You are not supposed to try to get rid of the thoughts and preoccupations at other times. Don't do anything, don't decide anything and don't think about anything at other times of the day. Just live your life as before and let things happen as they want. Next session, we can talk about it more.

Session Two

T: It is a pleasure to see you. So, tell me what you did with the exercises I asked you to do.

C: I stopped my medication that very same day. And I did the exercises. They were good, but hard to do, because I couldn't concentrate. And when I managed to bring them to my mind, I couldn't keep them there. They came and went. But the exercises were very effective, and my concentration has increased.

T: We will get to the exercises shortly. You said you stopped the medication. Was it easy for you to not take drugs anymore?

C: Yes, it was simple enough. And there weren't any after-effects. I just feel a little gloomy. Generally speaking, there was no problem.

T: Did you eat and sleep well during the week?

C: It was fine. I slept better, and I had less nightmares. I also ate well.

T: Now, you said that you did the exercises and they were effective. What do you mean by that?

C: Before beginning the exercises, my concentration was so low and I couldn't memorize what I'd studied. Having done the exercises, I feel that my mind has become free. I don't forget things as much as I used to, and I generally feel better.

T: Can you put your improvement in percentage terms?

C: I think I'm better by 30 or 40%.

T: Your second task was related to things. Tell me about it.

C: I did that too. I feel that I have greater control. Before this, when the ashtray occupied my mind, I immediately removed it from before my eyes. It's not like that anymore. It doesn't preoccupy me like that. My resistance has increased. Of course, I haven't completely overcome the power of things over me yet. They come every now and then and preoccupy my mind, but it's not as bad as it used to be.

T: How better is it?

C: I think the pressure related to things has decreased by 20 to 30%.

T: What about the couples?

C: I tested to see if I could concentrate or not through studying. I went to the library, and found couples. I started reading a newspaper while I paying attention to the couple. I felt I was able, to some extent, to get them out of my mind. But they still returned. I totally powerless against couples before, but after doing the exercises, I'm beginning to feel that I can exert some control over them.

T: Was a difference between things and people in your mind?

C: Imagining people was more difficult, and they came and went more often. But it was simpler about things.

T: I think you've made good progress. Here's what you are supposed to do for the rest of your treatment. Continue doing the exercise in this way: for the morning session (which was set to be at 8:00), recreate thoughts and preoccupations about couples for 5 min, and then allocate the other 5 min to the sexual fantasies. Recreate and re-experience the sexual fantasies just as they deluge your mind involuntarily, arouse you and probably force you to engage in some sort of sexual behavior. For the second session, which will be held at 19:00, recreate thoughts and preoccupations about couples for 5 min and follow it with another 5 min of recreating thoughts about things. At night, before going to bed, allocate the first 5 min to sexual fantasies.

Session Three

T: It's nice to see you again. Please tell me what you did.

C: I was able to do the exercises to some extent and the obsessive thoughts about couples and things do not bother me anymore. When I see two people together, I stop thinking about them the minute they move out of my sight. I can focus now. Before this, they kept entering my mind and made me lose concentration. And I no longer care about things, and I don't obsess over things around me.

T: In general, thoughts about things have left.

C: More or less.

T: And thoughts about couples have decreased.

C: Yes.

T: What about your sexual fantasies?

C: Sexual fantasies don't arouse me anymore. I no longer see women naked. During the exercises, no matter how I tried to imagine them naked, they kept appearing to me as clothed!

T: I asked you to imagine them as being naked, sexy and arousing. However, you could only imagine them wearing clothes, is that right?

C: Yes, it has become difficult to imagine them naked.

T: As I understand it, you have exams nowadays, and you need to focus on your studies. Has your studying improved?

C: When I start studying, I'm no longer preoccupied with things and people. However, I don't feel happy and satisfied. I feel bad. My past experiences (mainly lost opportunities and bereavements) come to my mind and bother me. I don't study with love and attention. I just study to get good marks and pass courses. I feel that I have lost my old enthusiasm for studying.

T: What about medication? Do you take drugs, yet? Tell me about it.

C: I no longer take drugs. Since yesterday, though, I've been feeling agitated, impatient and distraught. I am restless and I easily get angry and anxious.

T: Here's what you have to do up until next session: during the morning session (at 10:00) recreate thoughts about couples for 5 min. During the evening session (at 19:00) recreate the same thoughts for another 5 min. And at night, recreate sexual fantasies for 5 min before going to bed. The instructions are the same. Now, please tell me more about the restlessness and agitation.

C: When I think about lost opportunities, I feel upset and desperate and I feel restless and agitated. But if I think positively, and I forget about the past, it's almost as if I have no problems at all.

T: That's it?

C: Yes.

T: Well, if that is all about the restlessness and agitation, we need to add one more exercise to your previous tasks. For two sessions everyday (at 10:00 and 19:00), follow the first 5 min with another 5 min allocated to thoughts about lost opportunities in the past. Therefore, each session will amount to 10 min. You will recreate thoughts about the past similar to your other exercises. You must recreate those thoughts in such a way as to feel that the world has come to its end. You must recreate your worst mood possible.

C: Doctor, there is another problem too. Since these problems started (8 years ago) I haven't been able to maintain my friendship with my friends and my classmates. I can no longer have normal, close relationships with others.

T: Let us deal with this problem after your personal mood has improved.

Session Four

T: Pleasure to meet you again. Please tell me what you did.

C: I did the exercises regularly, except for certain days when I overslept.

T: Well, what was the result?

C: I have improved. I am no longer preoccupied with thoughts about couples and things, and I'm not bothered by them. I can study now, but I feel my memory has become weaker. I only needed to study stuff once in order to memorize and learn them. Now, however, I must study something several times, and I still can't remember it as well as before.

T: Let us go through tings one by one. Tell me more about your thoughts about things.

C: Things aren't important to me anymore. They used to bother me a lot during studying, but they are not an issue now.

T: And thoughts about couples?

C: They are very rare. They come and go like shadows.

T: Shadows?

C: They are not complete. They don't have bodies. It's just a shadow that moves past.

T: What about the sexual fantasies?

C: They have completely gone away. Now, when I see women in the streets, I see them as they are, not naked.

T: And bitter thoughts about the past?

C: They still bother me most of the time.

T: Last session, you told me about your restlessness and agitation. How have you been during the past two weeks?

C: I'm neither better nor worse.

T: You need to do another 5-min exercise (at 10:00) for recreating the remaining shadows of the couples. This time, you just focus on the shadows, not the actual couples. As for the restlessness, if they do not decrease gradually and they keep bothering you, you can ask your psychiatrist to prescribe medication just for these moods, in a low dose and for a short time.

As for the problem with your memory and learning your lessons, there are certain things you need to know. You've been dealing with serious problems for eight years, and you've been taking drugs for four years. These create special difficulties for you. So you must not expect your mind to be immediately as active and healthy as before. Right now, you are in the condition to engage in high mental labor and intensive studies. I understand your situation, the pressure will dwindle. You must decrease serious mental work for a year or two. You cannot expect your memory to work as well as when you were much younger, hadn't taken so much medication and did not have the problems you're dealing with now. You must not try to memorize any lessons. Your mind is not supposed to work like a clock right now. Just try to pass your exams, and remain healthy. We will visit in two years. Then, we can decide what needs to be done according to your condition.

21.3 Assessment of Treatment Outcome and Follow-Up

The course of the treatment was completed in 4 sessions. Assessment of the treatment outcome, which was based on the patients' comments in a graded scale of 0–100 and an open-ended question, indicated 80% recovery. A 35-month follow-up evaluation showed no relapse.

22 Client #20 (Female, 23 Years Old, Single)

22.1 Case Introduction

Miss. AK 23 years old student, was referred to the University of Tehran Clinic complaining about hair-pulling, difficulty impulse control, and her interpersonal (personality) problems. Her hair-pulling coupled with repeated intrusive and distressing thoughts that she will die soon started at the age of 12. The problems continued a couple of years, then she felt okay for about four years till the first year of her college. Since she entered the university, hair-pulling behavior came back more seriously. AK was diagnosed to have hair-pulling disorder based on DSM-5 accompanied by some degrees of impulse control disorder and interpersonal conflicts. The problems gradually got worse leading her to take medications for some times but AK stopped taking medication as she felt they were useless. This is her first visit to receive a psychological treatment. AK was seen for 4 sessions over a period of 6 weeks.

22.2 Course of Treatment

Session One

Therapist (T): (After greetings and the social stage of the interview) Please tell me why you have come here.

Client (C): I developed a habit of pulling my hair out when I was in the 6th grade. It went on for a couple of years. At the same time, I was really scared of death and heights. I remember I was in the 7th grade, and I always heard somebody telling me "you'll die in 10 or 15 min". And I really felt like I was about to die in 10 to 15 min. I couldn't breathe. Or I felt somebody telling me "don't eat this food; it's poisoned." There was always somebody with me. "Wash your hands several times. Because if you wash them only once, something bad will happen to you," it would say. I always had such thoughts. Time went by, and I got better upon entering high school. I didn't pull my hair out anymore. I was fine for four years. Then, my stress returned due to university and my new life (*the patient described her stress completely and was given a thorough explanation of pathological personality characteristics*); and with it came back the habit of pulling my hair out. It wasn't so bad at the beginning, but it gradually got worse and has been with me ever since.

T: Do you only pull the hair on your head, or do you do it with other parts of your body as well?

C: No, it's just the head. But it's gotten so severe, I can't stop doing it for even a second. I visited a psychiatrist, and I took medication for some time, but it was useless. So I stopped taking the drugs. I used to take drugs when I was a teenager, but that didn't help at all.

T: Under what circumstances does the pulling get worse, and when does it decrease?

M. A. Besharat, *Paradoxical Psychotherapy: A Practitioner's Guide*, University of Tehran Science and Humanities Series, https://doi.org/10.1007/978-3-031-27717-7_22

C: It doesn't decrease, it only gets worse when I'm stressed. The minute I start thinking about something, my hands move toward my head and I start pulling.

T: Do you just pull the hair out? Or do you, perhaps, eat it as well?

C: No, I just pull them out.

T: How do you sleep and eat?

C: They're fine, in general. I stay awake late at nights (until around 3:00 or 4:00), and then I oversleep till noon. I eat normally, but I eat a lot more when I'm stressed.

T: For now, we make a schedule based upon the pulling problem. You have to do some tasks according to my instructions. Here's what you need to do: on a specific time during the day (which we will agree upon shortly), you must engage in the habit of pulling your hair out for 5 min. Several times during the day, you pull your hair out involuntarily and compulsively. This unintentional pulling comes with certain emotions, and you are in an agitated, nervous mood. Now, your mood during the voluntary, pre-determined tasks must completely match how you feel in an uncontrolled frenzy of pulling. In each task, you must voluntarily recreate the compulsion, pressure, agitation and emotional state that you are thrown into at other times. If you can do each task in this way, you will get the best outcomes. There is, however, the possibility that you cannot make the task resemble your original emotional state by 100%, despite your honest attempts to do so; you only manage to recreate those feelings by 50%. You don't have to worry if such a thing happens, because you have made your best effort. The task might even be radically different from the real experience of pulling your hair out. But it doesn't matter either, as long as you have made an honest effort. On the other hand, keep in mind that the task must be done on fixed occasions. If you happen to be asleep during the time assigned to the task, or you are outside, or busy or cannot do it for any other reason, you must simply wait for the next occasion assigned for doing the task. You should not, under any circumstances, do the task at a time other than the occasions we will decide here. You simply lose the opportunity to do the task, and it doesn't matter. Actually, this losing is part of the treatment process. Now, I want you to consider your daily activities and then give me two times during the day when you can do the tasks. You will start tomorrow.

C: At 15:00 and 21:00.

T: There is something you must know. Your instruction is to do your task on these two occasions, starting tomorrow. I don't expect you to not pluck your hair out at other times, neither do I want you to try and stop plucking, or delay it in any other way. Whenever the involuntary urge comes to you to pull your hair out, just let it come and go. Don't try to stop it, and don't worry about it in any way. You only need to do your task on the two occasions in an optional and controlled manner. Whatever happens at other times, you can tell me about in the next session.

Session Two

T: It's nice to see you. You were supposed to do some tasks. Please tell me what you did.

C: I did the task for a week, and it was really interesting to me, since I didn't feel like pulling my hair out during the assigned times. I felt the same way all through the week, and I simply couldn't pull my hair, and I did it much less than before. After a week, I gave up doing the tasks, and the pulling returned last week.

T: You mean you did the tasks for only a week?

C: Yes.

T: The pulling decreased during that week, then you gave up the tasks and the pulling returned. I didn't limit the task to only a week, but perhaps you thought you must do it for just one week?

C: Yes, and we were supposed to have a session before the New Year, which was cancelled.

T: That's true. Unfortunately the New Year holidays delayed our second session. That's all right. Do the same task for two more weeks according to the following instruction: three 5-min occasions (P: At 10:00, 15:00 and 21:00) every day for the first week, and only on even days for the second week. The other instructions for doing the tasks are the same as what I told you in the first session.

Session Three

T: Nice to meet you. Please tell me what you did.

C: I did some of the pulling tasks, and I couldn't do all of them. I sat down on the assigned times, but I couldn't make myself pull a single strand of my hair. I didn't pull any hair at other times during the past two weeks.

T: You didn't pull any hair at all, or you pulled less than before?

C: I didn't pull any hair at all during the past two weeks.

T: How do you feel now that you don't pluck your hair out?

C: (Laughing) I'm so happy I can control myself; specially because there were times when I felt stressed, yet I didn't pull any hair out. There is another problem, though.

T: What?

C: I feel that I have become too sensitive when visiting my friends (my same-sex friends). I want them to pay attention to me. I have become more sensitive about what they say. I have become so irritable. I keep arguing with them, and we have quarrels all the time.

T: Actually, it is a good problem (the patient laughs). We will find a solution to it later on. Right now, we must remain focused on the pulling hair problem. Up to the next session, which is in two weeks, do the task once a day for 5 min. When can you do it?

C: At 22:00.

T: See you in two weeks.

Session Four

T: Nice to see you again. Tell me what you did.

C: I don't pluck my hair out anymore.

T: You didn't pull any hair during the past two weeks?

C: No, not at all.

T: Did you do the tasks?

C: Not so much, because I simply couldn't bring myself to pull my hair. I didn't feel the urge to pull them.

T: With respect to the pulling problem: we are now at a point when you have been able, for several weeks, to refrain from plucking your hair out. We have no other tasks for this problem. From now on, we need to work more on the personal issues you discussed earlier. As time goes by, we will know how completely the plucking problem has been treated. Since we cannot start the treatment of other problems right away, if the pulling habit comes back to you in the future, first let a couple of days pass. If the habit persists, you can arrange on your own a timetable similar to what I scheduled for you. Just be careful to do exactly what we did together: you agree to do the task three times a day, each time for 5 min. You should try to pull your hair out during these times. If you do it right, what happened here, will happen there as well. It may even happen faster and easier. Good luck!

22.3 Assessment of Treatment Outcome and Follow-Up

The course of the treatment was completed in 4 sessions. Assessment of the treatment outcome, which was based on the patients' comments in a graded scale of 0–100 and an open-ended question, indicated 100% recovery. A 25-month follow-up evaluation indicated that there was no relapse.[1]

[1] Hair-pulling disorder usually comes with problematic personality characteristics, and is usually accompanied with the impulse control disorder. For this reason, the treatment of impulse control disorder and other problematic personality characteristics must be taken into account when it comes to such cases, so that the possibility of relapse decreases.

23 Ending the PTC Treatment

The relationship between the therapist and the client is a short-term one in the PTC psychotherapy. The two sides must be ready to say goodbye soon. With the emergence of the first sings of ego-strength in the patient, the therapist must lead the treatment to its ending point. The coach (therapist) must believe in the player's (client) skills and send him/her to the field to compete against the rival (the disorder). The two-week and four-week intervals between the sessions don't allow the client to develop an attachment bond and or become dependent to the therapist. Therefore, it is not difficult to say goodbye. How does the treatment come to an end? In other words, how does the therapist announce the end to the treatment process? Relying on the progress made by the patient, the therapist says "I'm glad you've been able to overcome your problems through your own efforts. There is no more need for my direct supervision and guidance. We say goodbye at this point. In case you need to talk in the future, you can make an appointment. I do not think it will be necessary. You only need to keep certain points in mind." This is an example of how the therapist can end the treatment.

The points that have to be kept in mind: we ask the patient to do a minimum number of exercises for some time, and decrease them gradually. For instance, if the number of exercises before the last session has been once a day, the client is asked to do them once a day for one more week, and then decrease them to every other day during the second week. After that, the client no longer needs to do the exercises and must stop them. If the client has been doing the exercises every other day before the last session, he/she is asked to stick to the same timetable for one more week. Then, he/she must do the exercise two times during the next week (the days and the times for doing the exercises must be predetermined). Finally, he/she must cease doing the exercises from the third week.

Some of the advantages of concluding the treatment in this way are as follows: (1) the therapist trusts the patient's abilities and gives him/her the responsibility for his/her treatment. How would you feel if you are the patient and the therapist trust you in this way? (2) Removing the psychological distance between the therapist and the patient from the beginning of the treatment process. When the PTC therapist begins treatment with the intention of giving the client the responsibility for his/her own treatment, he/she is removing the distance between him/herself and the client. This therapist's attitude will have a definitive influence on forming rapport, making a genuine adaptation to the patient, having a live experience of the disorder, and adopting a neutral therapeutic stance; (3) removing the need for diagnosis, which is one of the characteristics of the PTC model; (4) complying with professional moral standards; (5) decreasing treatment expenses, both for the patient and for public health system.

M. A. Besharat, *Paradoxical Psychotherapy: A Practitioner's Guide*,
University of Tehran Science and Humanities Series,
https://doi.org/10.1007/978-3-031-27717-7_23

23.1 The Relapse

Predicting relapse is an important principle in the PTC model. The relapse rate in the PTC model is the lowest rate among all the psychotherapeutic methods. This has been proven experimentally (clinical and experimental recorded and videotaped evidence) and has scientific bases (both pathological and clinical).[1] Whether the patient mentions the possibility of relapse or not, the therapist offers the following explanation: "You will not suffer from this disorder/problem any more. However, in case a similar problem presents itself someday, first let a number of days pass. There is the possibility that the problem goes away after a few days. If, after a few days (usually five consecutive days), the problem does not go away, it's time for you to take action. Now, you have access to the formula for defeating this opponent. It is a simple formula you have used during your treatment here, and which you cannot forget. On the fifth day, you will draw a timetable for yourself to do the exercise from the next day for three x-minute times (the amount of time is defined according to the specific conditions of each patient). The same thing that happened under my supervision will happen again. This time, it will happen faster and more easily. This means that you won't need to come here again. Although, you are welcome here anytime you need."

23.2 The Roles of the Therapist and the Client in the PTC Model

Although the PTC model is applied under the supervision and guidance of the therapist, and the therapist plays an important role in managing the sessions and using interventions, it is a client-oriented treatment in terms of its outcomes (i.e., therapeutic changes). The central role of the PTC therapist is to remove the link between anxiety and the symptoms. That is all. Giving tasks, in terms of defining the nature of the task and doing them, is depended upon the patient. The patient plays a autonomous and active role in doing the paradoxical timetable, which consists of the simplest tasks the patient has ever encountered in his/her life. Through doing the exercises, the patient can believe in his/her capability for controlling the situations and playing a constructive role in treating him/herself. Such self-confidence acts as a strong barrier against relapse in the PTC model. When this self-confidence is couple with a simple therapeutic method (PTC), a method that can be used by the patient him/herself, its efficiency increases even more. In the PTC model, the therapist and the patient are not that far away from one another. They share rather similar roles. At some point during the treatment, the patient becomes completely independent of the therapist and turns into his/her own therapist.

23.3 Ten Questions for Further Thinking

I hope that reading the present book has been able to form huge questions in your mind. Are the following ten questions among the ones you have asked yourself? Do you want to think more about them? Do you know their answers?

1. What is a psychological disorder (mental illness)? Where does it come from? Where does it go? What purpose does it serve?
2. What role and responsibility does the patient assume with respect to the symptoms, therapeutic changes and the PTC therapist?
3. What stance does the PTC therapist adopt with respect to the patient, the symptoms and the treatment outcomes?
4. What is the therapeutic essence to the PTC model?
5. What is prescribed by the therapist for the patient in the paradoxical timetable?

[1] Other than the evidence provided by clinical and experimental data, some of which have been mentioned in the present book, and several other recorded ad videotaped evidence available at the author's clinical archives, the ego-strength, which is formed through the treatment process, is the main factor that prevents relapse. Refer to *The theoretical foundations of PTC: A perfect model of psychotherapy* (Besharat, 2023b).

6. What is the difference of increasing the dosage (the frequency of exercises) with the first and the second complements?
7. Why is the PTC model considered as a perfect psychotherapeutic model?
8. What kind of characteristics and behaviors on the parts of the therapist and the patient can act as barriers to treatment in the PTC model?
9. What position/value do ethics, law and economy occupy in the PTC model?
10. Do you think you can be a genuine PTC therapist after reading the present book, without needing to be trained, to do internships, and to receive supervisions?

Bibliography

Adler A (1923) The practice and theory of individual psychology. Routledge and Kegan Paul, London

Akillas E, Efran JS (1995) Symptom prescription and reframing: should they be combined? Cogn Ther Res 19:263–279

Allyon T (1963) Intensive treatment of psychotic behavior by stimulus satiation and food reinforcement. Behav Res Ther 1:53–62

American Psychiatric Association (2013) Diagnostic and statistical manual of mental disorders, fifth edition (DSM-V). American Psychiatric Publishing, Washington DC

Besharat MA (2018) PTC perfect model of therapy with couples: a practical guide. Tehran, Roshd Press. [Farsi]

Besharat MA (2023a) The principles of interviewing in PTC. Tehran, Psychoanalysts Press. [Farsi- in press]

Besharat MA (2023b) Theoretical foundations of PTC. Psychoanalysts Press, Tehran. [Farsi-in press]

Besharat MA (2023c) Paradox therapy for personality disorders-I: a practical guide. Psychoanalysts Press, Tehran. [Farsi]

Besharat MA, Naghipoor M (2019a) The application of a new model of paradox therapy for the treatment of illness anxiety disorder: a case report. Clin Case Rep Int 3:1–3

Besharat MA, Naghipoor M (2019b) Paradox therapy for the treatment of social anxiety disorder: a case study. J Syst Integr Neurosci 6:1–5

Besharat MA, Naghipoor M (2022) The application of paradox therapy for the treatment of obsessive-compulsive disorder: a case study. J Clin Case Rep Stud 3(4). https://doi.org/10.31579/2690-8808/106

Bateson G (1955) A theory of play and fantasy. Psychiatric Research Reports 2:39–51

Crowe M, Ridley J (2000) Therapy with couples: a bihavioural-systems approach to couple relationship and sexual problems. Blackwell Science, Oxford

Dinkmeyer DC, Pew WL (1979) Adlerian counselling and psychotherapy. Brooks/Cole, Monterey

Doherty WJ (1985) Values and ethics in family therapy. Counselling and Values 30:3–8

Dunlap K (1928) A revision of the fundamental law of habit formation. Science 67:360–362

Erickson MH (1959) Further clinical techniques of hypnosis: utilization techniques. Am J Clin Hypn 2:3–21

Erickson MH (1964) An hypnotic technique for resistant patients: the patient, the technique, and its rationale in field experiments. Am J Clin Hypn 7:8–32

Erickson MH (1965) The use of symptoms as an integral part of psychotherapy. Am J Clin Hypn 8:57–65

Erickson MH (1973) Psychotherapy achieved by a reversal of the neurotic process in a case of ejaculation praecox. Am J Clin Hypn 15:217–222

Erickson MH (1977) Hypnotic approaches to therapy. Am J Clin Hypn 20:20–23

Evans J (1980) Ambivalence and how to turn it to your advantage: adolescence and paradoxical intervention. J Adolesc 3:273–284

Frankl V (1939) Paradox intention. Schweiz Arch Neurol Psychiatry 43:26–31

Frankl VE (1973) Psychotherapy and existentialism: selected papers on logo therapy. Pelican Books, UK

Frankl VE (1991) Paradoxical intention. In: Weeks GR (ed) Promoting change through paradoxical therapy. Brunner/Mazel, New York, pp 99–110

Haley J (1963) Strategies of psychotherapy. Grune and Stratton, New York

Haley J (1984) Ordeal therapy: unusual ways to change behavior. Jossey Bass, San Francisco

Hull C (1943) Principles of behavior. Appleton, New York

Kraupl Taylor F (1969) Prokaletic measures derived from psychoanalytic techniques. Br J Psychiatry 115:407–409

MacIntyre AA (1987) Short history of ethics. Routledge and Kegan Paul, London

Madanes C (1981) Strategic family therapy. Jossey Bass, San Francisco

Mahoney MJ (1986) Paradoxical intention, symptom prescription, and principles of therapeutic change. Couns Psychol 14:283–290

Maranhao T (1984) Family therapy and anthropology. Cult Med Psychiatry 8:225–279

Marks IM (1970) The origin of phobic states. Am J Psychother 24:652–676

M. A. Besharat, *Paradoxical Psychotherapy: A Practitioner's Guide*,
University of Tehran Science and Humanities Series,
https://doi.org/10.1007/978-3-031-27717-7

Marks IM (1972) Flooding (implosion and related treatments). In: Agras WS (ed) Behaviour modification: principles and clinical application. Little Brown, Boston, pp 179–180

Papp P (1980) The Greek chorus and other techniques of paradoxical therapy. Fam Process 19:45–57

Selvini-Palazzoli M, Ceccin G, Prata G, Boscolo L (1978) Paradox and counterparadox. Jason Aronson, New York

Watzlawick P, Beavin J, Jackson D (1967) Pragmatics of human communication. W. W. Norton, New York

Watzlawick P, Weakland J, Fisch R (1974) Change: principles of problem formation and resolution. W. W. Norton, New York

Weeks GR, L'Abate L (1982) Paradoxical psychotherapy: theory and practice with individuals, couples and families. Brunner/Mazel, New York

Whan M (1983) Tricks of the trade: questionable theory and practice in family therapy. Br J Soc Work 13:321–327

GPSR Compliance
The European Union's (EU) General Product Safety Regulation (GPSR) is a set of rules that requires consumer products to be safe and our obligations to ensure this.

If you have any concerns about our products, you can contact us on

ProductSafety@springernature.com

In case Publisher is established outside the EU, the EU authorized representative is:

Springer Nature Customer Service Center GmbH
Europaplatz 3
69115 Heidelberg, Germany

www.ingramcontent.com/pod-product-compliance
Lightning Source LLC
Chambersburg PA
CBHW081222251125
35899CB00005B/87
* 9 7 8 3 0 3 1 2 7 7 1 6 0 *